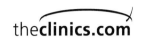

# SURGICAL CLINICS
# OF NORTH AMERICA

## Topics in Organ Transplantation for General Surgeons

GUEST EDITOR
Paul E. Morrissey, MD

CONSULTING EDITOR
Ronald F. Martin, MD

October 2006 • Volume 86 • Number 5

**SAUNDERS**

An Imprint of Elsevier, Inc.
PHILADELPHIA   LONDON   TORONTO   MONTREAL   SYDNEY   TOKYO

**W.B. SAUNDERS COMPANY**
*A Division of Elsevier Inc.*

1600 John F. Kennedy Blvd., Suite 1800, Philadelphia, PA 19103-2899

http://www.theclinics.com

| | |
|---|---|
| **SURGICAL CLINICS OF NORTH AMERICA** | **Volume 86, Number 5** |
| October 2006 | **ISSN 0039–6109** |
| Editor: Catherine Bewick | **ISBN 1-4160-3915-5** |

The ideas and opinions expressed in *The Surgical Clinics of North America* do not necessarily reflect those of the Publisher. The Publisher does not assume any responsibility for any injury and/or damage to persons or property arising out of or related to any use of the material contained in this periodical. The reader is advised to check the appropriate medical literature and the product information currently provided by the manufacturer of each drug to be administered to verify the dosage, the method and duration of administration, or contraindications. It is the responsibility of the treating physician or other health care professional, relying on independent experience and knowledge of the patient, to determine drug dosages and the best treatment for the patient. Mention of any product in this issue should not be construed as endorsement by the contributors, editors, or the Publisher of the product or manufacturers' claims.

*Surgical Clinics of North America* (ISSN 0039–6109) is published bimonthly by Elsevier Inc., 360 Park Avenue South, New York, NY 10010-1710. Months of publication are February, April, June, August, October, and December. Business and Editorial Offices: 1600 John F. Kennedy Blvd., Suite 1800, Philadelphia, PA 19103-2899. Customer Service Office: 6277 Sea Harbor Drive, Orlando, FL 32887-4800. Periodicals postage paid at New York, NY and additional mailing offices. Subscription prices are $385.00 per year for Institutional, $315.00 per year for Institutional USA, $385.00 per year Institutional Canada, $260.00 per year Personal, $200.00 per year Personal USA, $245.00 per year Personal Canada, $130.00 per year Personal student, $100.00 per year Personal student USA, $130.00 per year Personal student Canada. To receive student/resident rate, orders must be accompanied by name of affiliated institution, date of term, and the *signature* of program/residency coordinator on institution letterhead. Orders will be billed at individual rate until proof of status is received. Foreign air speed delivery is included in all *Clinics* subscription prices. All prices are subject to change without notice. POSTMASTER: Send address changes to *Surgical Clinics*, Elsevier Periodicals Customer Service, 6277 Sea Harbor Drive, Orlando, FL 32887-4800. **Customer Service: 1-800-654-2452 (US). From outside of the US, call 1-407-345-1000.**

*The Surgical Clinics of North America* is also published in Spanish by McGraw-Hill Interamericana Editores S.A., P.O. Box 5-237 06500 Mexico D.F. Mexico; and in Portuguese by Interlivros Edicoes Ltda., Rua Comandante Coelho 1085, CEP 21250, Rio de Janeiro, Brazil; and in Greek by Paschalidis Medical Publications, Athens Greece.

*The Surgical Clinics of North America* is covered in *Index Medicus, EMBASE/Excerpta Medica, Current Contents/Clinical Medicine, Current Contents/Life Sciences, Science Citation Index,* and *ISI/BIOMED.*

Printed in the United States of America.

# CONSULTING EDITOR

**RONALD F. MARTIN, MD,** Staff Surgeon, Department of Surgery, Marshfield Clinic, Marshfield, Wisconsin; Clinical Associate Professor of Surgery, University of Vermont, Burlington, Vermont; Lieutenant Colonel, United States Army Reserve, Medical Corps

# GUEST EDITORS

**PAUL E. MORRISSEY, MD,** Associate Professor of Surgery, Division of Organ Transplantation, Brown Medical School, Rhode Island Hospital, Providence, Rhode Island

# CONTRIBUTORS

**ROY K. AARON, MD,** Professor of Orthopaedics, Department of Orthopaedics, Brown Medical School, Providence, Rhode Island

**DEBORAH McK. CIOMBOR, PhD,** Associate Professor of Orthopaedics, Department of Orthopaedics, Brown Medical School, Providence, Rhode Island

**CHRISTOPHER J. COSGROVE, MD,** Clinical Assistant Professor of Medicine, Division of Nephrology, Transplant Section, Rhode Island Hospital, Providence, Rhode Island

**DAVID ELWOOD, MD,** Fellow in Liver Transplantation, Division of Hepatobiliary Surgery and Liver Transplantation, Lahey Clinic Medical Center, Burlington, Massachusetts

**STACI A. FISCHER, MD, FACP,** Assistant Professor of Medicine, Brown Medical School; Chief, Transplant Infectious Diseases, Rhode Island Hospital, Providence, Rhode Island

**AMITABH GAUTAM, MD,** Assistant Professor of Surgery, Division of Organ Transplantation, Brown Medical School, Rhode Island Hospital, Providence, Rhode Island

**REGINALD Y. GOHH, MD,** Associate Professor of Medicine (Nephrology), Division of Renal Diseases, Rhode Island Hospital, Brown University School of Medicine, Providence, Rhode Island

**DOUGLAS A. HALE, MD, FACS,** National Institute of Diabetes, Digestive, and Kidney Diseases, Transplantation Branch, National Institute of Health, Bethesda, Maryland

**NATHANIEL JELLINEK, MD,** Assistant Professor, Department of Dermatology, Brown Medical School, Rhode Island Hospital, Providence, Rhode Island

**KEVAN G. LEWIS, MD, MS,** Dermatology Resident, Department of Dermatology, Brown Medical School, Rhode Island Hospital, Providence, Rhode Island

**SONIA LIN, PharmD,** Clinical Associate Professor of Pharmacy, Department of Pharmacy Practice, College of Pharmacy, University of Rhode Island, Kingston, Rhode Island

**JOREN C. MADSEN, MD, DPhil,** Associate Professor of Cardiac Surgery, Transplantation Biology Research Center and Division of Cardiac Surgery, Department of Surgery, Massachusetts General Hospital, Harvard Medical School, Boston, Massachusetts

**ANTHONY P. MONACO, MD,** Professor of Surgery, Harvard Medical School, Beth-Israel Deaconess Medical Center, Boston, Massachusetts

**PAUL E. MORRISSEY, MD,** Associate Professor of Surgery, Division of Organ Transplantation, Brown Medical School, Rhode Island Hospital, Providence, Rhode Island

**CHOO Y. NG, MD,** Chief Resident in Cardiac Surgery, Transplantation Biology Research Center, Massachusetts General Hospital, Harvard Medical School, Boston, Massachusetts

**JAMES J. POMPOSELLI, MD, PhD, FACS,** Associate Professor of Surgery, Division of Hepatobiliary Surgery and Liver Transplantation, Tufts Medical School, Lahey Clinic Medical Center, Burlington, Massachusetts

**LESLIE ROBINSON-BOSTOM, MD,** Associate Professor, Department of Dermatology and Department of Pathology, Brown Medical School, Rhode Island Hospital-APC 10, Providence, Rhode Island

**GREG WARREN, DO,** Fellow in Nephrology, Rhode Island Hospital, Brown Medical School, Providence, Rhode Island

**MATTHEW J. WEISS, MD,** Resident in General Surgery, Transplantation Biology Research Center, Massachusetts General Hospital, Harvard Medical School, Boston, Massachusetts

**JAMES WHITING, MD,** Associate Professor of Surgery (Transplantation Surgery), Maine Medical Center, Division of Organ Transplantation, Portland, Maine

# CONTENTS

Humans are protected from a daily onslaught of pathogenic organisms by an immune system that provides multiple layers of protection. Until solid organ transplantation became technically feasible in the early twentieth century, this constant state of surveillance for foreign cells that are associated with the immune response mostly was viewed as advantageous. Unfortunately for patients who have end-stage failure of the heart, lungs, kidney, liver, and pancreas, the immune system is incapable of distinguishing between the presence of beneficial foreign tissue and harmful foreign pathogens; it mounts an effective attack against both. Improving our understanding of the factors that initiate and perpetuate the alloimmune response will result in the development of more refined and better tolerated immunosuppressive strategies.

The requirement for immune suppression after solid organ transplantation increases the risk of infection with a myriad of organisms. There are many unique and evolving aspects of infection after solid organ transplantation. Advances in immunosuppressive therapy and improved protocols for infection prophylaxis have resulted in changes in the timing and clinical presentation of opportunistic infections. Vigilance in the diagnostic evaluation of suspected infection in the solid organ transplant recipient is essential. This article reviews the basic evaluation and treatment options for many of the infectious conditions peculiar to the immunosuppressed patient.

## The Preoperative Evaluation of the Transplanted Patient for Nontransplant Surgery

Reginald Y. Gohh and Greg Warren

With the improved success of solid-organ transplantation, there has been an increased willingness to transplant individuals previously felt to be unsuitable for such procedures. Factors such as age and various medical comorbidities are no longer considered contraindications to transplantation, and hence, an increasing number of recipients may require medical care not specifically related to the transplant. After transplantation, many of these patients may require elective or emergent surgery, making it important for all surgeons to be familiar with the factors that may influence surgical outcomes in this population, as well as factors that affect postoperative care. Most transplant centers use a team approach to manage these complex patients, relying on medical professionals experienced in their care and management. Close interaction with the transplant team is likely the single most important step in preparing the transplanted patient for surgery and managing their postoperative care.

## Perioperative Management of Immunosuppression

Sonia Lin and Christopher J. Cosgrove

Current immunosuppressive regimens typically consist of two phases: induction phase (medications given at the time of the initial transplant) and maintenance therapy. Induction medications are given to decrease the occurrence of early acute rejection, avoid or minimize corticosteroids, and potentially induce long-term favorable immunoregulatory effects. As tolerance remains an elusive goal, life-long maintenance immunosuppression is required after all solid-organ transplantations. The various agents used in these two phases of immunosuppression are reviewed in this article. The similarities and differences between the agents within each class, with respect to efficacy and tolerability, are discussed.

## Perioperative Concerns for Transplant Recipients Undergoing Nontransplant Surgery

James Whiting

At some time in a general surgeon's career it is likely that they will be asked to care for a surgical problem in a transplant recipient. In many instances, the treating surgeon may opt for transferring the patient to a transplant center more familiar with organ transplant recipients, but at other times transfer may not be the optimal option for the patient. This article is intended to touch on some of the more common situations that a general surgeon in community practice might encounter in dealing with organ transplant recipients, and highlight perioperative and in a few cases, intraoperative, concerns.

## Gastrointestinal Complications Following Transplantation

Amitabh Gautam

Gastrointestinal complications are common after kidney, liver, pancreas, heart, and lung transplantation. Complications can include gastrointestinal conditions preceding the transplantation, viral, fungal, and bacterial gastrointestinal infections, and gastrointestinal side effects of medications including immunosuppressive agents. Establishing the etiology of gastrointestinal complaints is often difficult because any one or a combination of these factors might be contributory in the same patient.

## Hepatobiliary Surgery: Lessons Learned from Live Donor Hepatectomy

David Elwood and James J. Pomposelli

The liver is unique in that rapid tissue regeneration occurs after resection or injury, and affords the surgeon the opportunity to safely remove up to 60% to 70% of the liver volume for treatment of cancer or for use as a live donor graft for transplantation. The complex development of the liver and biliary system in utero results in multiple and complicated anatomic variations. The hepatobiliary surgeon of today must be able to integrate a broadening array of radiologic and liver resection techniques that may improve patient safety and surgical outcome. Equally important is the ability to quickly recognize postoperative complications so that prompt intervention can be instituted. Successful outcome requires a balance between sound judgment, technical acumen, and attention to detail. Herein, we provide lessons learned from live donor liver transplantation that are directly applicable to any patient undergoing major hepatic resection.

## Living Kidney Donation: Evolution and Technical Aspects of Donor Nephrectomy

Paul E. Morrissey and Anthony P. Monaco

For more than 40 years, living donor nephrectomy was performed through a flank incision drawn on the urologic experience with nephrectomy for cancer. Since its introduction one decade ago, laparoscopic donor nephrectomy has gained widespread acceptance and popularity; currently over one-half of donor nephrectomies in the United States are performed with this technique. The changing practice of donor nephrectomy resembles in many ways the evolution of minimally invasive surgery in other subspecialties. The lessons learned from these technical developments are valuable and can be adapted by general surgeons and urologists when called upon to perform nephrectomy for organ donation or kidney disease.

# FORTHCOMING ISSUES

**December 2006**

**Surgical Critical Care**
Juan Carlos Puyana, MD and Matthew Rosengart, MD, *Guest Editors*

**February 2007**

**Trauma**
Ronald V. Maier, MD, *Guest Editor*

# RECENT ISSUES

**August 2006**

**Recent Advances in the Management of Benign
and Malignant Colorectal Diseases**
Robin P. Boushey, MD, PhD,
and Patricia L. Roberts, MD, *Guest Editors*

**June 2006**

**Surgical Response to Disaster**
Robert M. Rush, Jr, MD, *Guest Editor*

**April 2006**

**Current Practice in Pediatric Surgery**
Mike K. Chen, MD, *Guest Editor*

**February 2006**

**Evidence-Based Surgery**
Jonathan Meakins, MD and Muir Gray, MD, *Guest Editors*

**December 2005**

**Perioperative Issues for Surgeons**
Lena Napolitano, MD, *Guest Editor*

---

## The Clinics are now available online!

### www.theclinics.com

SURGICAL
CLINICS OF
NORTH AMERICA

Surg Clin N Am 86 (2006) xi–xiii

# Foreword

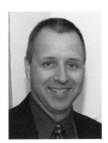

Ronald F. Martin, MD
*Consulting Editor*

I am deeply indebted to Dr. Paul Morrissey and his colleagues for producing this issue on topics relating to transplantation for the general surgeon. There are a multitude of reasons for general surgeons to have an interest in "transplantation-related" topics, many of which are found within the confines of this issue. If from reading this issue a practicing surgeon were only to glean a better understanding of the physiologic changes of the transplantation patient or to have a better understanding of the infectious, gastrointestinal, or neoplastic considerations some of these patients develop, I would consider this issue a success. Yet there is much more to learn from the transplantation community at large. Dr. Morrissey and his colleagues would probably be too humble to list the lessons we can learn from them, so I shall take the liberty of commenting on some of the lessons we could—and, in my opinion, should—learn from our colleagues.

Transplantation surgeons are the hardest working and most dedicated group of physicians that I know of. Most of them work in teams, and for the most part those teams are highly functional despite long hours and arduous tasks. The emphasis on teamwork and de-emphasis on individual behavior amongst and between transplant physicians, surgeons, and nonsurgeons alike, is largely responsible for the tremendous success their discipline has enjoyed in the past several decades.

Transplantation centers and physicians tend to colocate their service facilities and personnel. Even in highly competitive markets, cooperation is as likely to be found as competitive behavior. To be certain, there are "boutique" transplantation programs and there are competitive transplantation

doi:10.1016/j.suc.2006.08.007                    *surgical.theclinics.com*

programs and physicians. Furthermore, some degree of "cooperation" may be imposed by external regulation. Yet the transplantation community largely exhibits a defined focus and agenda and shares information and technology. By centralizing programs, which are labor-, finance-, and resource-intensive (to say the least), the transplantation community has shown what I think should be a fundamental tenet of modern health care: transportation of the patient with complex needs to centers with a critical mass of services and personnel is almost invariably less expensive and more successful than unnecessary duplication of resources.

Nearly all of our transplantation programs are actively involved with clinical and basic science investigation. The research provided by their endeavors has provided us all with useful information for the "nontransplant" patient, particularly in the critically ill, or those suffering from infectious disease. The long tradition of inquiry in the transplantation field is, of course, well recognized and is exemplified by one of our American colleagues, Dr. Joseph Murray, who received the Nobel Prize for his contributions to human kidney transplantation. The transplantation community leads our profession in developing and maintaining databases and exhibiting transparency of those databases to one another as well as the government and the public in general. In times when a desire is being well verbalized by third-party payers, governmental organizations, public interest groups, and health care "purchasing" consortiums for access to our performance and outcome data, we could all benefit from the lessons of the transplantation community.

The transplantation community is perhaps the only segment of our profession that has really had to deal with rationing of health care resources—though I suspect if there was an oversupply of donor organs or bioartificial devices, there may be an unlimited number of procedures performed, just as in the rest of the field. Regardless of this speculation, there is a limited supply of organs, and as such a system has been created to determine how to best determine which patients will derive the greatest benefits from which organs. One could argue the validity of scoring systems or the net result of organ allocation or that the living related donor system invalidates the model, but one would be hard-pressed to argue that the transplantation community has not at least begun to address the fundamental question of modern health care in our nation: What is the *value* of a service not only to the individual, but also to society? Few, if any, of the rest of us have to make that decision (outside of the mass casualty or disaster model) for and with our patients. Furthermore, the model for determining value has evolved as the technology, resources, and outcomes have evolved.

Lastly, our transplantation colleagues show an unparalleled commitment to their patients; their willingness to engage in any problem of their patient, whether transplantation-related or otherwise, is widely known and recognized. This may or may not be a "good" lesson as we strive to develop more efficient overall health care delivery systems, but it is certainly an admirable trait.

The *Surgical Clinics of North America* series continues to deliver information that is of interest and applicability to any general surgeon. Although an extremely small subset of surgeons will ultimately be responsible for performing an organ transplantation or managing that patient's care afterward, most of us are likely to participate in the care of a patient who has undergone organ transplantation or will soon need to. Hopefully this issue will be of help to you in such times.

Ronald F. Martin, MD
*Department of Surgery*
*Marshfield Clinic*
*1000 North Oak Avenue*
*Marshfield, WI 54449, USA*

*E-mail address:* martin.ronald@marshfieldclinic.org

ELSEVIER
SAUNDERS

Surg Clin N Am 86 (2006) xv–xvii

SURGICAL
CLINICS OF
NORTH AMERICA

# Preface

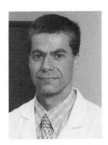

Paul E. Morrissey, MD
*Guest Editor*

On December 23, 2004, clinical transplantation celebrated its 50<sup>th</sup> anniversary. After decades of experimental efforts in animal and human transplantation the first successful solid organ transplant was performed between identical twins. The recipient became the first survivor of end-stage renal disease in world history. By the start of the next decade, rudimentary hemodialysis and renal transplantation from deceased and nontwin living donors were available. Subsequent improvements in immunosuppression and innovative efforts of many surgeons enabled successful transplantation of the heart, liver, pancreas, lung, and small bowel. The success of these programs led to a proliferation of transplants that was unimaginable even 20 years ago. Administered through the United Network of Organ Sharing, which is awarded the federal contract to oversee deceased donor transplantation from the Organ Procurement and Transplantation Network (http://www.optn.org/), transplantation in the United States now includes some 258 certified programs within 58 organ procurement organizations. Last year, 28,110 solid organ transplantations were performed in the United States; 6895 of these were coincident with procurement from a living donor. Because the allograft half-life is greater than 10 years for many organs, the number of patients with a functioning transplant is rapidly rising. As a result, it is increasingly likely that general surgeons will be called to care for a transplant recipient from time to time.

doi:10.1016/j.suc.2006.08.006

*surgical.theclinics.com*

This issue seeks to provide a resource for general surgeons to answer the following questions:

- What special considerations are required when caring for transplant recipients?
- What are the current immunosuppressive regimens and how might they affect surgical care?
- What lessons can be applied from transplantation to general surgical practice?
- What does the future hold for transplantation?

The articles in this issue fall into several categories, beginning with immunobiology and ending with a look toward the future of organ transplantation. In between these scientific discussions are several articles pertaining to the preparation of the transplantation patient for general surgery; two articles on surgical techniques used for liver and renal transplantation that can be adapted to general surgical practice and two articles highlighting common complications of immunosuppression that might be encountered by the practicing general surgeon (skin cancer and bone disease). Transplantation immunobiology remains unfamiliar, perhaps even mystical, to most general surgeons. The articles in this text are understandable and straightforward. Basic principles are emphasized, but so is the redundancy of the immune system such that an appreciation of its underlying complexity is acquired. The authors have done a tremendous job of tackling a difficult subject matter and distilling it to a digestible story, which demystifies and informs rather than overwhelms. The clinical articles are intended to be practical. The material could be read for basic knowledge and later serve as a reference for patient care. Finally, the surgical techniques can be incorporated into the general surgeon's armamentarium for preoperative planning for partial liver resections or anterior approaches to the retroperitoneum.

In preparing this issue of the *Surgical Clinics of North America*, I have used individuals recognized for their outstanding contributions in transplantation. Each is an established educator in transplantation. A broad group of authors from pharmacy, research, medicine, and surgical subspecialties was selected to achieve balance in this issue. Their dedication to teaching and the practice of transplantation is obvious by their willingness to participate in this issue. Their commitment to this challenging group of patients is evidenced by the repeated admonition to involve the transplantation team in the general surgical care of transplant recipients.

It goes without saying that my family always provided me with encouragement and understanding affording me the time to take on this project. Their continued love and support made this project particularly enjoyable. I wish, if only informally, to dedicate this text to Anthony P. Monaco, MD, who has been my mentor in transplantation since my Fellowship years at the New England Deaconess Hospital in Boston. He has served as a teacher and advisor to many of the authors who are featured in this issue, and their participation is a testimonial to his exemplary practice over the years. I also wish to express my appreciation to Catherine Bewick at Elsevier for her helpful editorial assistance and guidance. Finally, I offer my gratitude to Ron Martin, MD, who developed the concept for this issue—a collection of transplantation reviews that are relevant and meaningful to the practicing surgeon. I hope that we have achieved this goal and in doing so have provided a useful reference for general surgeons who care for patients after solid organ transplantation.

Paul E. Morrissey, MD
*Division of Organ Transplantation*
*Rhode Island Hospital*
*593 Eddy Street, APC 921*
*Providence, RI 02903, USA*

*E-mail address:* pmorrissey@lifespan.org

ELSEVIER
SAUNDERS

SURGICAL
CLINICS OF
NORTH AMERICA

Surg Clin N Am 86 (2006) 1103–1125

# Basic Transplantation Immunology

## Douglas A. Hale, MD*

*Room 5-5-750, Building 10, 10 Center Drive, Transplantation Branch,
National Institute of Diabetes & Digestive & Kidney Diseases,
National Institutes of Health, Bethesda, MD 20892, USA*

Ever since complex forms of life first appeared on earth, they have been under a near constant state of attack from environmental pathogens. This extraordinary evolutionary pressure has culminated in the development of multiple complex biologic defense mechanisms that, when combined, make up the human immune system [1]. This complexity is reflected in the overall structure of the immune system and, just as importantly, in its control. Regarding its structure, the immune system is organized in a tiered fashion and presents a formidable defense in depth by responding to the threat of foreign pathogens in a continually escalating fashion. Accordingly, threats are met first with simple barrier functions, which, if not successful in neutralizing the threat, are superseded by simple, nonspecific phagocytic functions. If these fail similarly to contain the proliferative capacity of the invading organism, progressively more specific and augmented responses are elicited until the foreign pathogen prevails or is destroyed.

At the risk of oversimplification, before initiating an attack the immune system must make two determinations. First, it must detect that the offending organism is foreign or nonself. Second, it must determine a context for the encounter with the foreign organism (ie, does the foreign tissue pose a threat?). Ideally, the immune system would recognize that an organ allograft is foreign tissue that represents no threat and would fail to mount a response. Unfortunately, such is not the case. Consequently, the immune system initiates a variety of attack strategies that must be offset pharmacologically for the transplanted organ to survive.

---

Preparation of this manuscript was supported by intramural funding through the National Institutes of Health.

* University of Florida, Jacksonville Transplant Center at Shands, 580 West 8th Street, # 8000, Jacksonville, FL 32209.

*E-mail address:* Douglas.Hale@jax.ufl.edu

Because the immunologic response to an organ allograft bears many similarities to the response that is directed against foreign pathogens, this article seeks to provide nontransplant surgeons with an appreciation of the general organization and function of the human immune system. Some specific immunologic consequences of allotransplantation, the practical implications of this knowledge, and the theoretic basis of modern immunosuppression are addressed subsequently.

## Cells and organs of the immune system

The functional cells of the immune system arise from hematopoietic stem cells and can be divided into those that are derived from myeloid or lymphoid precursors. Both precursors can give rise to a variety of cells within their established lineage.

Granulocytic cells of myeloid origin can be classified as being neutrophils, eosinophils, or basophils, depending upon their particular cytoplasmic staining characteristics and cellular morphology. Generally, neutrophils are the first cells to arrive at a site of inflammation. They develop in the bone marrow and migrate to the circulating blood for a few hours until they make their way into the tissues. Neutrophils contain granules that are packed with substances which, when released upon contact with a pathogen, are responsible for killing the target cell. Eosinophils are much like neutrophils in that they are motile phagocytic cells. They differ from neutrophils in that their granules stain with eosin and their phagocytic activity is aimed predominantly at parasitic organisms. Unlike neutrophils and eosinophils, basophils possess no phagocytic function. Instead they contain granules that release pharmacologically active compounds during certain types of allergic reactions.

The mononuclear cell population is represented by monocytes in the peripheral blood and macrophages in the tissue. Monocytes develop from myeloid progenitors in the bone marrow, are released into the bloodstream for a brief period of time, and then migrate into tissues and differentiate into macrophages. Depending upon in what tissue they reside, macrophages can assume several roles. Macrophages are the primary cells that are responsible for the digestion and destruction of foreign pathogens.

Dendritic cells are specialized cells of myeloid origin that are so named because they possess long filamentous-like processes that resemble the dendrites of nerve cells. They are located strategically in tissues with a high probability of encountering foreign antigen. As will be seen later, they play a crucial role in the initiation of the adaptive immune response.

Cells that are derived from lymphoid precursors can be characterized broadly as T lymphocytes (T cells), B lymphocytes (B cells), and natural killer (NK) cells. They can be discriminated from one another by their characteristic expression of certain surface molecules. B cells were so named based upon early observations that they derive from an organ called the bursa of the Fabricius in birds. In humans, B cells develop and mature in the bone marrow, and can be characterized by the expression of membrane-bound immunoglobulin. Once activated, they evolve into plasma cells and secrete antibody that possesses roughly the same specificity as that previously expressed on the membrane. T cells can be differentiated from B cells in that they possess receptors that are capable of discriminating self cells from non-self cells. T cells originate in the bone marrow but mature during their passage through the thymus. They can be divided into helper T cells (characterized by the expression of the CD4 surface molecule) and cytotoxic T cells (characterized by the expression of the CD8 surface molecule). In general, the role of helper T cells is to recognize a foreign threat and then secrete various cytokines to orchestrate the destruction of the threat. Conversely, the predominant role of the cytotoxic T cell is to respond to cytokines that are secreted by the helper T cells by releasing toxins that result in the destruction of the cells that constitute the threat. NK cells are unique in that they do not express surface molecules that are capable of recognizing a specific antigen. Instead, these cells possess activating receptors that are capable of recognizing complement fragments and antibodies coating the target cell surface. In addition, to prevent a direct attack on one's own tissues, these cells possess a receptor that inhibits activation when a NK cell comes into contact with a self cell.

The secondary lymphatic tissues provide anatomic support for the function of the cellular components of the immune system. Lymph nodes are numerous, small, bean-shaped structures that are integral components of the lymphatic drainage system. They contain large numbers of lymphocytes and are organized in such a fashion so as to maximize the likelihood of a productive interaction between the contained lymphocytes, as well as foreign antigens and antigen-presenting cells that are contained in the lymph. The spleen serves an analogous role for hematogenously drained foreign antigen. The thymus is the primary site for early selection, maturation, and education of T cells. It is here that T cells with high avidity or low avidity for self tissues are deleted through active and passive processes, respectively. As a result, autoimmunity and ineffectual immunity are prevented.

## Distinguishing self from nonself

Insofar as the human immune system exists to protect the host from foreign threats, it is incumbent to understand just what it is that renders humans immunologically unique from potential pathogens and, by extension, from one another. Human beings, in most cases, are distinguishable from one another based upon a repertoire of major and minor histocompatibility antigens that are encoded by the major histocompatibility complex (MHC) in their genome and expressed as HLAs on their cell membranes.

Major histocompatibility antigens are divided into three classes: class I, class II, and class III with the class I and class II antigens being most relevant for purposes of our discussion. These antigens are encoded within a continuous segment of DNA on chromosome 6 in humans. The loci that constitute the MHC are highly polymorphic (ie, many alternative forms of each gene exist). Each individual inherits a set of antigens from each parent. As a result, each individual expresses two distinct sets of MHC molecules that render him or her distinct from most other humans.

Class I and class II MHC molecules facilitate the recognition of foreign cells by binding, what is in most cases, small peptide fragments that are derived from processed proteins that originate from the foreign pathogens and presenting them to host T cells. Class I MHC molecules are expressed on most human tissues. The mechanism whereby peptides are bound to class I of molecules stipulates that most peptides that are presented by class I MHC molecules originate within the cell itself. As a consequence, class I molecules typically present endogenous self peptides as well as intracellular peptides that are associated with pathologic conditions, such as viral infections or tumor antigens. MHC class II molecules are expressed more selectively on populations of cells that typically are involved in stimulating an immune response in the role of antigen-presenting cells (macrophage, dendritic cell, B cell). In addition, their expression can be induced in a broad array of tissues during an injury response. In contrast to MHC class I molecules, MHC class II molecules predominately present peptides that originate outside of the cell and which are endocytosed, processed, and bound.

By virtue of their distinct molecular structures, MHC class I and class II molecules further distinguish themselves by interacting with characteristically distinct lymphocyte populations. For example, MHC class I molecules typically interact with T-cell receptors that are associated with the CD8 molecule (cytotoxic T cell). In contrast, MHC class II molecules typically interact with T-cell receptors that are associated with the CD4 molecule (helper T cell).

### Innate immune system

For purposes of organization, the human immune system is composed of two fundamentally different, but functionally interrelated, components. These are the innate and adaptive immune systems. The innate immune system is characterized by the fact that it is nonspecific and possesses no mechanism for the establishment of immunologic memory. Insofar as it is capable of reacting in an immediate fashion, the innate immune system generally is responsible for providing the initial defensive barrier and cellular response against foreign organisms.

After the physical barrier represented by the skin and mucous membranes, the tissue phagocytes represent the next line of defense against foreign pathogens (Fig. 1). One type of tissue phagocyte, the macrophage, evolves from a circulating monocyte and migrates into tissues throughout the body. Neutrophils are the second major type of tissue phagocyte present and are found predominantly in the blood. Both phagocytic cells play a major role in the innate immune response because they are capable of

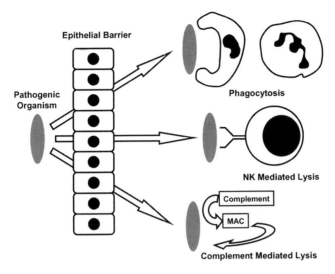

Fig. 1. Components of the innate immune system. The skin and mucous membranes provide anatomic barrier protection against foreign pathogens. Once the barriers have been breached, nonspecific phagocytic and cytotoxic activity is provided by tissue phagocytes (eg, macrophages, granulocytes) and NK cells. Molecules on the cell membrane of foreign pathogens also can activate the cytotoxic complement cascade directly. MAC, membrane attack complex.

recognizing and destroying foreign pathogens independently of the adaptive immune response. Neutrophils and macrophages can discriminate between pathogens and normal host tissue through membrane-bound receptors that recognize carbohydrate residues (ie, mannose) or lipopolysaccharides that typically are expressed on pathogens. The binding of a phagocyte to a pathogen through these receptors results in the phagocytosis of the pathogen. The initial interaction between the macrophage and the pathogen also results in the secretion by the macrophage of a host of proinflammatory molecules, such as prostaglandins, leukotrienes, and platelet-activating factor. This action is responsible for initiating an inflammatory process that culminates in the further recruitment of neutrophils and macrophages to the site of injury.

The complement system also plays a crucial role in the recognition of pathogens by the innate immune system [2]. The complement system consists of a large number of inactive precursor plasma proteins that interact with one another through an activation cascade that results in the production of peptides that are capable of coating the surface of the pathogen. These peptides also can bind simultaneously to receptors that are present on phagocytic cells, and, thereby, facilitate the process of phagocytosis. Other soluble complement proteins that are released during the activation cascade serve as chemotactic factors by attracting leukocytes to an area of inflammation. The classic pathway of complement activation can be initiated directly through the binding of the first protein in the complement cascade, C1q, to the pathogen. Alternatively, the spontaneous hydrolysis of the complement protein C3 on the pathogen's surface can result in activation of the complement cascade. This is termed the alternative pathway for complement activation. In addition to producing numerous small complement fragments as byproducts of the cascade activation process, the terminal products of the cascade assemble into a membrane attack complex that is capable of creating a pore in the lipid bilayer membrane of a pathogen, which destroys its structural integrity. The classic pathway also can be activated by the binding of C1q to antibody molecules that are bound to antigens, and, thus, create an antigen antibody complex (see later discussion). Thus, the complement system plays a crucial role in the innate and adaptive immune responses that are discussed later.

Similar to complement, NK cells serve effector functions in the innate and adaptive immune response and can serve as a bridge between both arms of the immune system [3,4]. Although ultimately they are of lymphoid origin, they differ from T and B cells in that they do not possess antigen-specific receptors. NK cells home to an area of inflammation through the influence of chemokines and cytokines that are released by activated macrophages and possess many types of receptors, most of which have functions that remain to be elucidated. Two types of receptors have been characterized well, however, and they consist of a stimulatory receptor that recognizes a wide variety of conserved pathogen-associated molecular patterns that are present on many organisms, and an inhibitory receptor that is specific for self MHC class I molecules. In this manner, noninfected cells can resist attack by NK cells. Alternatively, because infected cells exhibit reduced MHC class I expression, they are less capable of inhibiting an attack by NK cells that have been activated.

Despite its limitations, the innate immune system serves as a reliable first responder against foreign pathogens. Its major strength in this regard is its rapid onset of activity. The major weaknesses of the innate immune response are its lack of specificity, which can lead to excessive destruction of local tissues, a limited potential for amplification, and its failure to develop immunologic memory. These deficiencies are addressed through the subsequent activation of the adaptive immune response.

## Afferent limb of adaptive immune response

Although activation of the innate immune response may be sufficient for dealing with minor threats, major threats persist despite its best efforts. In this case, the major benefit derived from the innate response is that it can inhibit the rate of progression of the threat while the adaptive response is mounted. In addition, cytokines that are released by cells that participate in the persisting innate response serve as stimulation for the adaptive response.

The recognition phase of the adaptive immune response, although influenced by the processes of inflammation and the innate immune response, formally begins with the interaction between a CD4$^+$ T cell and a professional antigen-presenting cell (Fig. 2). Antigen-presenting cells can be of myeloid (ie, macrophage, dendritic cell) or lymphoid (B cell) lineage. Upon activation, these cells typically are capable of expressing high levels of class II MHC molecules and other accessory molecules that are necessary for initiation of an immune response. Activation of antigen-presenting cells typically occurs following exposure to foreign antigen and substances (ie, interferon [IFN]-γ or lipopolysaccharide) that are released by cells participating in the innate immune response.

Successful initiation of an adaptive immune response is believed to depend upon three major signals being delivered to the T cell. First, antigen-specific recognition occurs through engagement of the T-cell receptor with processed foreign antigen in the context of a self MHC class II molecule. A second signal, termed a costimulatory signal, serves to lower the activation threshold of the T cell [5]. Although a variety of costimulatory pathways has been described, the best characterized ones involve the lymphocyte membrane-bound molecules CD154 and CD28 and the cognate ligands CD40 and CD80/CD86. Upon activation, expression of CD40 and CD80/CD86 molecules is increased in antigen-presenting cells, which increases the likelihood of a successful interaction between it and a T cell. The recognition of foreign antigen presented in the context of self MHC

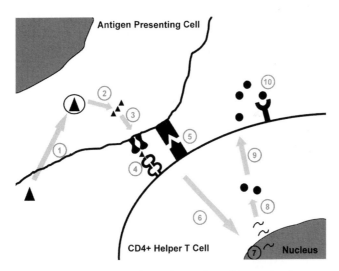

Fig. 2. Recognition phase of adaptive immunity consists of interaction between an antigen-presenting cell (APC) and T helper cell. (1) Foreign antigen is taken up by the APC. (2) The foreign antigen is processed into peptide fragments. (3) Peptide fragments are loaded onto MHC class II molecules and presented on the cell surface. (4) Foreign peptide and self MHC are recognized by the T cell receptor. (5) Binding of costimulation molecules present on the APC and T cell occurs. (6) Signal transduction pathway results in production of transcription factors for IL-2 and other cytokines. (7) IL-2 transcripts are produced and (8) translated. (9) IL-2 is released and (10) binds to CD25, which results in T-cell proliferation.

and simultaneous ligation of costimulatory molecules results in the production of interleukin (IL)-2 by the lymphocyte. Proliferation of the newly activated T cell is driven by the binding of IL-2 to its receptor CD25. Not surprisingly, once a lymphocyte begins the process of activation, CD25 expression is increased, which further ensures the effective initiation of the adaptive response.

## Efferent limb of adaptive immune response

There are multiple possible effector responses that can be elicited once the CD4+ T cell is activated by virtue of its interaction with an antigen-presenting cell (Fig. 3). The precise nature of the effector response that develops ultimately is determined by the immunologic milieu that is present during the time of this interaction.

The prototypical alloimmune effector response involves the generation and proliferation of cytotoxic CD8+ T cells. Cytotoxic T cells possess a T-cell receptor that is capable of recognizing foreign antigen in the context of self class I MHC. For a cytotoxic T cell to activate and attack a target cell, it requires help in the form of cytokines that are elaborated by helper

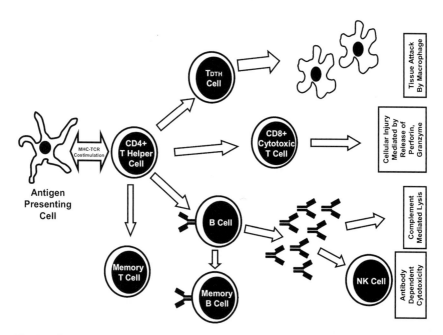

Fig. 3. Effector mechanisms of adaptive immunity. The interaction between the antigen-presenting cell and T helper cell results in the elaboration of cytokines that determine the nature of the effector responses. Conventional cytotoxicity and delayed-type hypersensitivity are two possible cell-mediated responses. Complement-mediated cytotoxicity and antibody-dependent cytotoxicity are two possible antibody-mediated responses. TCR, T-cell receptor.

T cells that also have been activated by an antigen-presenting cell in the same vicinity. The colocation of these processes is facilitated by the organization of the secondary lymphoid tissues. Once it has received sufficient stimulation, the cytotoxic T cell proliferates and is capable of releasing a variety of cytotoxic substances (ie, perforin, granzyme) upon its next encounter with cells that express the target antigen.

B cells recognize foreign antigen through its binding to the B-cell receptor. The B-cell receptor consists, in part, of membrane-bound antibody, all of which expresses the same specificity. Cross-linking of adjacent membrane-bound antibody molecules on the surface of the B cell by foreign antigen serves as the initial component of the recognition phase of B-cell activation. The antigen is internalized through a process that is known as receptor mediated endocytosis, and processed into peptide fragments. Simultaneously, cross-linking of membrane-bound antibody up-regulates the expression of MHC class II molecules and costimulatory molecules on the cell surface. The foreign antigen peptide fragments are loaded and presented on the MHC class II molecules where they are recognized by $CD4^+$ T cells. The up-regulation of costimulatory molecules on the B-cell surface facilitates T-cell activation, which results in the up-regulation of CD154 expression and its binding to the CD40 molecule on the B cell. This process, with additional assistance from the elaboration of cytokines by the T helper cell, drives B-cell proliferation, maturation into a plasma cell, and antibody production. The antibody that is produced by each plasma cell possesses roughly the same specificity as the original membrane-bound antibody component of the B-cell receptor that was present on the B cell that originally was activated.

Antibodies can cause damage through a variety of mechanisms. The predominant pathway through which antibodies mediate cellular injury is activation of the complement protein cascade. Complement activation can occur through the classic pathway following the formation of soluble antigen antibody complexes or following the binding of antibody to antigen on a suitable target, such as the bacterial cell wall or allograft tissue. Once the antibody binds to the antigen, conformational changes occur in the portion of the antibody molecule that is capable of binding to the C1 component of the complement system. Following this, a chain reaction is initiated that ultimately culminates in the production of a membrane attack complex. This complex disrupts the structure of membrane phospholipids and creates a large transmembrane channel that disrupts the integrity of the membrane of the target cell.

Alternatively, antibody can mediate damage through a process that is known as antibody-dependent cell-mediated cytotoxicity. Antibody molecules possess two sites that are specific for antigen and one site (Fc) that is capable of fixing complement. Several types of cells that have cytotoxic potential, such as macrophages, monocytes, neutrophils, and NK cells, express membrane receptors for this Fc region of the antibody molecule. Because of this, antibody can serve as a bridge between targeted pathogens and cytotoxic cells. Once the cytotoxic cell has been drawn to the target cell, it effects target cell killing through the elaboration of cytokines (ie, tumor necrosis factor [TNF]) or a variety of lytic enzymes.

Another important effector mechanism is termed delayed type hypersensitivity. This is a less specific form of immunologic attack than typically is associated with the adaptive immune response. In this process, the generation of specialized $CD4^+$ cells ($T_{DTH}$ cells) results in the elaboration of chemokines (ie, macrophage inhibition factor) and cytokines (IL-2, IFN-$\gamma$, TNF-$\beta$) that are capable of recruiting and activating macrophages. The macrophages develop increased phagocytic activity as a result. The activated macrophages then begin to attack and destroy cells in the local area; this results in destruction of the offending organism and, unfortunately, any surrounding inflamed host tissue.

In addition to the orchestration of immediate effector mechanisms, the adaptive immune response also results in the generation of long-lived T and B cells, also known as memory cells. Memory cells retain their original specificity and by virtue of their previous exposure to foreign antigen, have a lower threshold for subsequent activation and the capability to respond more rapidly. Their existence accounts for the observation of immunity following vaccination as well as the documented rapid marshalling of an immune response that follows repeated exposure to the same foreign antigen.

Finally, not all effector mechanisms of the adaptive immune response are oriented toward the destruction of the targeted threat. Instead, one particular mechanism is directed primarily at inhibiting the immune response in an antigen-specific fashion. This mechanism has been termed regulation and can be mediated by a variety of cells, but most notably by a subpopulation of $CD4^+$ T cells that is characterized by the stable expression of CD25 [6]. These cells, otherwise known as Treg cells, recognize foreign antigen in a fashion similar to other $CD4^+$ T cells. In contrast to conventional T helper cells, however, the local immunologic milieu at the time of this interaction results in the production of a Treg cell that produces cytokines (ie, TGF-$\beta$) or expresses surface molecules (CTLA4) that are capable of inhibiting the development of a cytotoxic response. This particular mechanism probably evolved to facilitate the termination of an immune response once it is no longer necessary and as an alternative means of controlling autoimmunity [7–9].

## The alloimmune response

Although their evolutionary purpose has been to protect the host from infectious pathogens, most of the effector mechanisms that were discussed in the previous section also can be directed against an allograft. This is in contrast to the early belief that the alloimmune response was predominantly a cytotoxic reaction that was mediated by $CD8^+$ cytotoxic T cells and orchestrated through cytokines elaborated by $CD4^+$ T helper cells. Although this particular effector pathway is important, it has become increasingly clear that other effector mechanisms, such as a humoral response, delayed type hypersensitivity, antibody-dependent cytotoxicity, and even the innate immune response, are capable of mediating substantial damage to the allograft. These similarities to the conventional immune response aside, because the immune system did not evolve specifically to frustrate the efforts of transplant surgeons, the artificiality of an allotransplant scenario does result in the observation of several phenomena that otherwise would not occur commonly in nature.

One of these atypical phenomena has to do with the mode of antigen presentation to the helper T cell, a crucial first step in the activation of the adaptive immune system (Fig. 4). Recipient helper T cells are capable of recognizing fragments of donor MHC molecules that have been processed by antigen-presenting cells of recipient origin (indirect pathway). Although this more closely resembles the naturally occurring processes that define a response against a foreign pathogen, this approach generally is believed to play a subservient role in producing an alloimmune response. Instead, recipient T cells also are capable of directly recognizing intact donor MHC on donor tissue and activating as a consequence of this interaction. This is termed the direct pathway of alloantigen recognition, because the donor antigen is not processed through self-antigen presenting cells. This mode of recognition seems to dominate the process of early immunologic engagement between the recipient and donor [10,11].

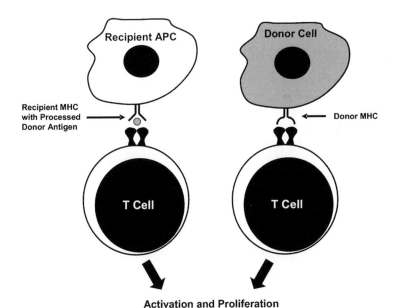

Fig. 4. Antigen presentation. Recipient T cells can recognize donor MHC molecules (especially on donor antigen-presenting cells [APCs]) directly in addition to being capable of recognizing processed donor antigen in the context of self MHC.

The alloimmune response also can be distinguished by the fact that it is associated with more injury and trauma at the outset than is a typical immune response against an infectious pathogen. The surgery that is necessary for the implantation of the allograft—combined with the inevitable injury that is associated with a transient period of ischemia, cold storage, and reperfusion—create a markedly proinflammatory environment that is ripe for eliciting a robust adaptive immunologic response [12]. In addition, ischemia-reperfusion results in the necrosis/apoptosis of some donor cells; this process can provide a potent stimulus for the activation of NK cells of the innate immune system through the release and expression of substances that can stimulate their Toll-like receptors [13,14]. In an effort to counteract this immunologically hostile environment, the current practice of transplant physicians is to administer the greatest amount of immunosuppression during the period of time immediately surrounding the time of transplant.

With the recognition that the immunologic response against an allograft is more broadly based that was appreciated previously, interest in humoral alloimmunity, in particular the development of antibody specific for donor HLA, has grown. Although early research has long suggested that the presence of antidonor antibody was associated with the development of chronic allograft injury [15], the full implications of the presence of antidonor antibody is just now becoming clear [16,17]. The major reason for the delay in appreciating the role of antidonor antibody in the alloimmune response was the absence of suitable assays that demonstrated a link between the two. The recent development of high throughput assays for anti-HLA antibodies [18], combined with the demonstration of a relationship between C4d deposition in allograft capillary walls (as demonstrated by way of immunohistochemistry) and the presence of anti-donor HLA antibodies [19], have provided this link. C4d is a split product that is released by the complement activation cascade; its presence strongly implicates the presence of antidonor antibody deposition because there are few other mechanisms available for activating the complement cascade in an allograft. Using these tools, the evidence supporting a major role for antidonor HLA antibodies in allograft loss has become compelling [20–23]. Consequently, major efforts are underway to develop effective therapies for controlling humoral immunity in transplant recipients.

Heterologous immunity represents another avenue that figures prominently in the production of a deleterious alloimmune response [24,25]. Effective immunologic reactions result in the production of cells that are capable of neutralizing that threat as well as a specialized population of long-lived memory T and B cells that serve to accelerate subsequent responses to the same antigen. Unfortunately, the specificity of these memory cells is not absolute, and as humans age they accumulate increasing numbers of these cells that, although initially specific for various previously encountered foreign antigens, also are cross-reactive toward donor antigen. These memory cells, having been primed already, are capable of responding against their original antigen and antigens that they are cross-reactive to more quickly and efficiently than when responding to an antigen for the first time [16,26]. These memory cells also are more resistant to the effects of modern immunosuppressive agents [27]; as a result, they represent a potent barrier to graft survival. These observations take on additional significance with the recognition that the number of T cells that is capable of recognizing and responding to allogeneic antigen exceeds—by several orders of magnitude—the number of T cells that normally is capable of responding to a naturally occurring antigen [28].

The specific role of the development of Treg cells that are capable of attenuating the adaptive immune response directed against an organ allograft is an area of active investigation. Some preliminary evidence suggests that the presence of donor-specific regulatory cells is associated with an improved outcome (ie, longer survival, less rejection) [29,30]. In addition, the impact of modern immunosuppressive regimens on the development of this cell population is just beginning to be appreciated [31,32]. Further investigation in this field seeks to determine how we can alter the management of early immunosuppression to maximize the generation of donor-specific Treg cells and, in so doing, minimize the requirement for long-term immunosuppression.

## Clinical applications of transplant immunology

### Maintenance immunosuppression

Maintenance immunosuppression consists of the drug or combination of drugs used chronically to prevent allograft rejection. Because the clinical application of immunosuppressive agents is covered in detail elsewhere in this issue, this section only provides background regarding the molecular mechanisms through which the commonly used agents act.

Because most of the early crucial steps of immune recognition and attack are mediated predominantly by lymphocytes, modern immunosuppressive drugs target pathways that are responsible for lymphocyte activation and proliferation (Fig. 5). Engagement of the T-cell receptor, combined with simultaneous binding of costimulation molecules, results in the activation of a signal transduction pathway that culminates in the production of IL-2. A key intermediate step in this pathway is the removal of a phosphate group from cytoplasmic nuclear factor of activated thymocytes, which then translocates to the nucleus where it is a transcription factor necessary for the production of transcripts for IL-2 and several other molecules. Tacrolimus and cyclosporine, mainstay agents in current use, bind to cytoplasmic proteins that are called immunophilins to form a complex that blocks the phosphatase activity of calcineurin. This prevents the formation and nuclear translocation of transcription factors that are necessary for the production of IL-2 transcripts. The end result is markedly impaired lymphocyte function.

Antiproliferative agents have played a role in immunosuppressive regimens since the original demonstration of their efficacy by Calne [33].

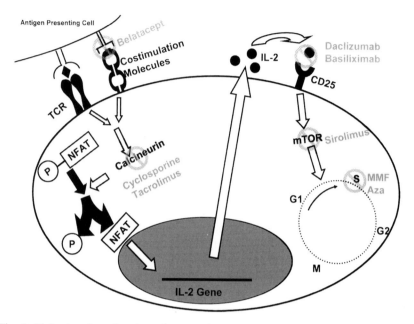

Fig. 5. Molecular sites of action of current immunosuppressive agents. Cyclosporine and tacrolimus bind to an immunophilin and this complex prevents the generation of nuclear factor of activated thymocytes (NFAT) by inhibiting the activity of calcineurin. Sirolimus bind to an immunophilin and then combines with mTOR. This complex inhibits cell cycle progression by blocking S6 kinase activity. MMF and azathioprine (AZA) inhibit lymphocyte proliferation by restricting the supply of guanosine available for DNA synthesis. Daclizumab and basiliximab block interaction between IL-2 and CD25. Belatacept blocks the interaction between CD28 on the T cell and CD80/CD86 on the antigen-presenting cell.

Lymphocytes, unlike many other cells, only can generate the building blocks of DNA through one pathway. These agents work by inhibiting lymphocyte proliferation by interfering with the synthesis of purines or pyrimidines. The two available agents in this class are azathioprine and mycophenolate mofetil (MMF). Azathioprine is metabolized to 6-mercaptopurine and subsequently to 6-ionosine monophosphate, a potent inhibitor of key enzymes in the de novo pathway of purine synthesis. MMF is metabolized to mycophenolic acid, which is a noncompetitive inhibitor of inosine monophosphate dehydrogenase. Both drugs result in depletion of guanosine nucleotides in T and B lymphocytes.

Sirolimus is an immunosuppressive agent that was discovered in the early 1970s, but it was not approved for clinical use until the late 1990s. Like cyclosporine and tacrolimus, sirolimus also binds to an immunophilin. Binding of the drug with its immunophilin results in the formation of an immunosuppressive complex by combining with mammalian target of rapamycin (mTOR) [34]. The sirolimus-immunophilin-mTOR complex inhibits activation of a S6 kinase that ultimately prevents progression of the cell cycle from G1 to S phase, and, by extension, blocks cellular proliferation [35].

Belatacept is an investigational monoclonal antibody that is being used in clinical trials. It selectively blocks binding of CD28 with CD80 or CD86, and prevents the costimulation signal that normally is provided through this pathway. A recent study demonstrated that when administered intermittently, belatacept could substitute effectively for cyclosporine in an immunosuppressive regimen that also included MMF and steroids [36].

*Induction immunosuppression*

Induction immunosuppression refers to the use of high doses of immunosuppression in the immediate peritransplantation time frame. The traditional goal of this therapy has been to minimize the risk for rejection during the period of time when the threat is highest. In its more commonly accepted form, it generally refers to the administration of biologic agents (ie, antibodies). In classic terms, induction immunosuppression consists of the administration of lymphocyte-depleting antibodies. Available agents can be categorized as being monoclonal (all antibodies have same specificity) or polyclonal (contains antibodies possessing a broad range of specificities).

OKT3 is a mouse IgG monoclonal antibody that is specific for the T-cell receptor that was introduced into clinical practice in the mid-1980s. OKT3 administration is associated with extensive T-cell depletion through a variety of mechanisms [37]. Binding of the OKT3 antibody to the ε chain of the CD3 membrane receptor of the T cell also can result in the internalization of the receptor antibody complex, which renders the T cell nonfunctional [38].

Polyclonal antilymphocyte globulin preparations have been used successfully as induction immunosuppression agents since their first reported use by Starzl and colleagues [39]. The agent that is used most often is a rabbit antihuman polyclonal antilymphocyte preparation. The predominant mechanism of activity is depletion of lymphocytes that are bound with the administered antibodies. This depletion is accomplished through a variety of mechanisms, including complement-mediated lysis, antibody-dependent cytotoxicity, activation-induced cell death, and apoptosis [40–42]. In addition to depletion of lymphocytes, polyclonal antithymocyte globulins contain a host of nondepletional, nonlymphocyte-specific antibodies that, nonetheless, have substantial potential for impacting the immunologic milieu [43–45].

Alemtuzumab (campath) is a humanized monoclonal antibody whose administration results in prompt elimination of the recipient's circulating lymphocytes [46]. It has a binding domain for CD52, which is expressed by essentially all T and B lymphocytes, and most monocytes, macrophages, eosinophils, NK cells, and dendritic cells [47]. There are three proposed mechanisms whereby alemtuzumab contributes to lymphocyte depletion: complement fixation, antibody-dependent cell-mediated cytotoxicity, and growth inhibition as a consequence of cross-linking the CD52 target antigen

[48–50]. When used as an induction agent, it has been successful in markedly reducing the requirement for maintenance immunosuppression [51].

Although lymphocyte depletion clearly can be related to a reduced risk for rejection in the early posttransplant period, one potential unfortunate consequence of lymphocyte depletion is homeostatic proliferation. This refers to the accelerated rate of proliferation of residual naive lymphocytes in a host rendered lymphopenic [52]. As a consequence of this proliferation, these cells can adopt a memory phenotype, even in the absence of encountering an antigen, and have a lower threshold for activation following a subsequent encounter with antigen [53]. The precise implications of this observation for long-term control of the alloimmune response are unclear at present.

Monoclonal antibodies that target the α chain of CD25 are relative newcomers to the induction immunosuppression armamentarium, and are effective in reducing the risk for rejection in the first 6 months following renal transplantation when combined with traditional maintenance immunosuppression [54,55]. The mechanism of activity seems to be mostly due to the inhibition of IL-2 binding to CD25, although some other mechanisms have been suggested [56,57].

*Tissue typing*

Because the immunologic reaction in solid organ transplantation is restricted largely to one direction (ie, recipient against donor), only the MHC molecules that appear different to the recipient's immune system are relevant to the study of transplant immunology. Instances in which donor MHC molecules differ from that of the recipient are termed mismatches. Because two MHC class I loci (A and B) and one MHC class II locus (DR) are analyzed routinely, and because each individual carries two alleles for each, a total of six possible mismatches is possible.

Kidney and pancreas allografts are assigned prospectively to individuals on the waiting list according to criteria emphasizing the length of time that they have been on the list, but also taking into account certain levels of mismatching of MHC alleles between the donor and recipient. This practice is based upon historical studies that suggested that a measurable survival benefit is associated with low levels of mismatching between the donor and recipient MHC specificities at the A, B, and DR loci [58]. Liver, heart, lung, and intestinal allografts are allocated without regard to degree of MHC mismatch, although the data are collected for retrospective analysis.

MHC typing can be accomplished using a variety of methods that can be classified as being high or low resolution. High-resolution, molecular-based methodologies can determine single amino acid differences between MHC molecules that otherwise appear identical using low-resolution polymerase chain reaction–based molecular assays or serologic testing. Low-resolution techniques suffice for purposes of solid organ transplantation; high-resolution sequencing is necessary for unrelated bone marrow transplantation.

*Crossmatch testing*

Previous encounters with cells that possess foreign MHC antigens, such as occurs as a consequence of blood transfusion, pregnancy, or previous transplant, can result in the production of long-lived memory B cells and the persistence of anti-MHC antibody. If an individual is transplanted with an organ that expresses MHC molecules for which they have pre-existing antibody, the antibody will bind to the endothelium of the organ allograft, activate complement and procoagulant cascades, and result in the near immediate loss of graft viability. This process has been termed "hyperacute rejection," and its incidence has been reduced markedly following the adoption of pretransplant crossmatching [59,60]. In crossmatching procedures, donor T and B cells are incubated with serum that is obtained from the recipient. If antidonor antibodies are present they bind to the donor cells and can be detected using a variety of methods. Pretransplant crossmatching is performed routinely for recipients of kidney and pancreas allografts. It also is performed selectively in recipients of heart transplants who are known to have increased levels of anti-MHC antibodies based upon screening tests that are done regularly while patients are awaiting an organ. Positive crossmatches in these scenarios preclude transplantation, and the organ would be allocated to an alternative recipient. Prospective crossmatching is not necessary for liver transplantation.

## Tolerance

The induction of donor-specific immunologic tolerance is a long sought after goal of transplantation researchers. Tolerance can be defined as a state characterized by the specific lack of unrestrained adverse immune reactivity, the maintenance of which does not require chronic immunosuppression. Given that the current 1-year graft survival for recipients of kidney, pancreas, or liver allografts is now in excess of 90%, some might wonder whether the potential benefit to be gained justifies the risk for clinical trials in this field [61]. Unfortunately, however, a chronic inexorable attrition in allograft survival occurs during the subsequent 4 years following transplantation, which results in 5-year graft survivals of approximately 75% or less [62]. In addition, even with the current refinements made to standard immunosuppressive regimens, including improved antimicrobial prophylaxis, the morbidity that is associated with nonspecific immunosuppression remains substantial.

Experimentally, tolerance can be induced by a variety of methods in rodent models and is maintained by multiple immunologic mechanisms. Although the rodent has been used historically to test various approaches of tolerance induction because it is characterized well immunologically, it has the major disadvantage of being generally more permissive for tolerance induction than are higher animal and human models. With this in mind, the two most promising approaches for tolerance induction that have been translated successfully to higher animal models from rodents include costimulation blockade and depletion/reconstitution (using donor marrow or stem cells).

The use of costimulation blockade to induce tolerance is a new development since it was demonstrated first that blockade of CD28 (using CTLA4Ig) in diabetic mice resulted in tolerance to human pancreatic islets [63]. When applied to nonhuman primate solid organ allograft models, long-term graft survival can result from short periods of drug administration; however, indefinite graft survival seems to require the chronic intermittent administration of the blocking agent [64,65]. Tolerance induction protocols that use costimulation blockade have not been tested widely in a human solid organ transplant model. A trial to evaluate the efficacy of CD40/CD154 blockade was halted early in its conduct because of thrombotic complications [66].

The use of donor bone marrow to facilitate tolerance induction traces it origin back to the original tolerance experiments that were conducted by Medawar, and it has been combined successfully with a variety of nonmyeloablative conditioning regimens (radiation, chemotherapy, depletional antibody, immunosuppression) [67]. In rodent models, the end result generally is a stable state of mixed chimerism (coexistence of donor and recipient bone marrow) and a robust state of tolerance. Generally, when this approach has been applied to higher animal solid organ allograft models, a transient low-level state of mixed chimerism is produced that persists for a month or two. The loss of chimerism does not seem to effect graft survival [68]. At the human level, there are many reported instances in which an individual who has undergone successful bone marrow transplantation has received a subsequent kidney allograft from the same individual that donated the marrow allograft [69]. In these instances, the recipient has been immunologically tolerant of the kidney allograft and chronic immunosuppression has not been required. Unfortunately, the efficacy, morbidity, and mortality that are associated with bone marrow transplantation make its general use as a tolerance induction regimen in solid organ transplantation unacceptable. Regimens that combine donor bone marrow or stem cells with less morbid forms of conditioning have not, despite a few successes, permitted the successful withdrawal of chronic immunosuppression on a consistent basis [70–76].

The induction of tolerance also has been attempted through the application of potent lymphocyte-depleting strategies at the time of transplant. Using a strongly depletional approach to tolerance induction, primates that were treated briefly with an anti-CD3 immunotoxin and deoxyspergualin demonstrated complete tolerance to kidney allografts and subsequent challenge grafts. Changes consistent with chronic rejection were not seen in these animals even after 5 years of observation, during which time no immunosuppression was administered [77–79]. Recent attempts to induce donor-specific hyporesponsiveness (if not tolerance itself) in humans using this approach generally have permitted a reduction in the amount of chronic immunosuppression that is required to prevent rejection, but have not permitted complete immunosuppression withdrawal [51,66,80,81].

## Summary

Refined through the application of millions of years of evolutionary pressures, the human immune system represents a formidable barrier to the long-term survival of organ allografts. Although the immune response against an organ allograft bears some similarities to a conventional response against a pathogenic organism, the unique circumstances that surround and follow the implantation of an organ transplant have resulted in the observation of previously unanticipated consequences. Nonetheless, recent advances in our understanding of transplant immunology have improved clinical outcomes sufficiently to justify widespread application of allotransplantation for many forms of end-stage failure of the heart, lung, liver, pancreas, and kidney. Continued investigation is indicated to refine our ability to control the antiallograft immune response and to reduce (and perhaps eventually eliminate) the need for chronic, nonspecific immunosuppression and its attendant morbidity.

## References

[1] Pancer Z, Cooper MD. The evolution of adaptive immunity. Annu Rev Immunol 2006;24: 497–518.

[2] Rus H, Cudrici C, Niculescu F. The role of the complement system in innate immunity. Immunol Res 2005;33(2):103–12.

[3] Young NT. Immunobiology of natural killer lymphocytes in transplantation. Transplantation 2004;78(1):1–6.

[4] O'Connor GM, Hart OM, Gardiner CM. Putting the natural killer cell in its place. Immunology 2006;117(1):1–10.

[5] Croft M, Dubey C. Accessory molecule and costimulation requirements for CD4 T cell response. Crit Rev Immunol 1997;17(1):89–118.

[6] O'Garra A, Vieira P. Regulatory T cells and mechanisms of immune system control. Nat Med 2004;10(8):801–5.

[7] Cassis L, Aiello S, Noris M. Natural versus adaptive regulatory T cells. Contrib Nephrol 2005;146:121–31.

[8] Raghavan S, Holmgren J. CD4$^+$CD25$^+$ suppressor T cells regulate pathogen induced inflammation and disease. FEMS Immunol Med Microbiol 2005;44(2):121–7.

[9] Wraith DC, Nicolson KS, Whitley NT. Regulatory CD4$^+$ T cells and the control of autoimmune disease. Curr Opin Immunol 2004;16(6):695–701.

[10] Jiang S, Herrera O, Lechler RI. New spectrum of allorecognition pathways: implications for graft rejection and transplantation tolerance. Curr Opin Immunol 2004;16(5):550–7.

[11] Illigens BM, Yamada A, Fedoseyeva EV, et al. The relative contribution of direct and indirect antigen recognition pathways to the alloresponse and graft rejection depends upon the nature of the transplant. Hum Immunol 2002;63(10):912–25.

[12] Land WG. The role of postischemic reperfusion injury and other nonantigen-dependent inflammatory pathways in transplantation. Transplantation 2005;79(5):505–14.

[13] Andrade CF, Waddell TK, Keshavjee S, et al. Innate immunity and organ transplantation: the potential role of toll-like receptors. Am J Transplant 2005;5(5):969–75.

[14] Olszewski WL. Innate immunity processes in organ allografting—their contribution to acute and chronic rejection. Ann Transplant 2005;10(2):5–9.

[15] Jeannet M, Pinn VW, Flax MH, et al. Humoral antibodies in renal allotransplantation in man. N Engl J Med 1970;282(3):111–7.

[16] McKenna RM, Takemoto SK, Terasaki PI. Anti-HLA antibodies after solid organ transplantation. Transplantation 2000;69(3):319–26.

[17] Terasaki PI. Humoral theory of transplantation. Am J Transplant 2003;3(6):665–73.

[18] Pei R, Lee J, Chen T, et al. Flow cytometric detection of HLA antibodies using a spectrum of microbeads. Hum Immunol 1999;60(12):1293–302.

[19] Feucht HE, Felber E, Gokel MJ, et al. Vascular deposition of complement-split products in kidney allografts with cell-mediated rejection. Clin Exp Immunol 1991; 86(3):464–70.

[20] Terasaki PI, Ozawa M. Predicting kidney graft failure by HLA antibodies: a prospective trial. Am J Transplant 2004;4(3):438–43.

[21] Michaels PJ, Fishbein MC, Colvin RB. Humoral rejection of human organ transplants. Springer Semin Immunopathol 2003;25(2):119–40.

[22] Michaels PJ, Espejo ML, Kobashigawa J, et al. Humoral rejection in cardiac transplantation: risk factors, hemodynamic consequences and relationship to transplant coronary artery disease. J Heart Lung Transplant 2003;22(1):58–69.

[23] Pelletier RP, Hennessy PK, Adams PW, et al. Clinical significance of MHC-reactive alloantibodies that develop after kidney or kidney-pancreas transplantation. Am J Transplant 2002;2(2):134–41.

[24] Adams AB, Pearson TC, Larsen CP. Heterologous immunity: an overlooked barrier to tolerance. Immunol Rev 2003;196:147–60.

[25] Taylor DK, Neujahr D, Turka LA. Heterologous immunity and homeostatic proliferation as barriers to tolerance. Curr Opin Immunol 2004;16(5):558–64.

[26] Adams AB, Williams MA, Jones TR, et al. Heterologous immunity provides a potent barrier to transplantation tolerance. J Clin Invest 2003;111(12):1887–95.

[27] Pearl JP, Parris J, Hale DA, et al. Immunocompetent T-cells with a memory-like phenotype are the dominant cell type following antibody-mediated T-cell depletion. Am J Transplant 2005;5(3):465–74.

[28] Sherman LA, Chattopadhyay S. The molecular basis of allorecognition. Annu Rev Immunol 1993;11:385–402.

[29] Salama AD, Najafian N, Clarkson MR, et al. Regulatory CD25$^+$ T cells in human kidney transplant recipients. J Am Soc Nephrol 2003;14(6):1643–51.

[30] Muthukumar T, Dadhania D, Ding R, et al. Messenger RNA for FOXP3 in the urine of renal-allograft recipients. N Engl J Med 2005;353(22):2342–51.

[31] Gregori S, Casorati M, Amuchastegui S, et al. Regulatory T cells induced by 1 alpha, 25-dihydroxyvitamin D3 and mycophenolate mofetil treatment mediate transplantation tolerance. J Immunol 2001;167(4):1945–53.

[32] Zheng XX, Sanchez-Fueyo A, Sho M, et al. Favorably tipping the balance between cytopathic and regulatory T cells to create transplantation tolerance. Immunity 2003;19(4): 503–14.

[33] Calne RY. The rejection of renal homografts. Inhibition in dogs by 6-mercaptopurine. Lancet 1960;1:417–8.

[34] Heitman J, Movva NR, Hall MN. Targets for cell cycle arrest by the immunosuppressant rapamycin in yeast. Science 1991;253(5022):905–9.

[35] Kuo CJ, Chung J, Fiorentino DF, et al. Rapamycin selectively inhibits interleukin-2 activation of p70 S6 kinase. Nature 1992;358(6381):70–3.

[36] Vincenti F, Larsen C, Durrbach A, et al. Costimulation blockade with belatacept in renal transplantation. N Engl J Med 2005;353(8):770–81.

[37] Bonnefoy-Berard N, Revillard JP. Mechanisms of immunosuppression induced by antithymocyte globulins and OKT3. J Heart Lung Transplant 1996;15(5):435–42.

[38] Galante NZ, Camara NO, Kallas EG, et al. Modulation of peripheral blood T-lymphocytes in kidney transplant recipients treated with low dose OKT3 therapy. Immunol Lett 2004; 91(1):75–7.

[39] Starzl TE, Marchioro TL, Hutchinson DE, et al. The clinical use of antilymphocyte globulin in renal homotransplantation. Transplantation 1967;5(4):(Suppl):1100–5.

[40] Genestier L, Fournel S, Flacher M, et al. Induction of Fas (Apo-1, CD95)-mediated apoptosis of activated lymphocytes by polyclonal antithymocyte globulins. Blood 1998;91(7): 2360–8.

[41] Lenardo M, Chan KM, Hornung F, et al. Mature T lymphocyte apoptosis—immune regulation in a dynamic and unpredictable antigenic environment. Annu Rev Immunol 1999;17: 221–53.

[42] Michallet MC, Saltel F, Preville X, et al. Cathepsin-B-dependent apoptosis triggered by antithymocyte globulins: a novel mechanism of T-cell depletion. Blood 2003;102(10): 3719–26.

[43] Bonnefoy-Berard N, Vincent C, Revillard JP. Antibodies against functional leukocyte surface molecules in polyclonal antilymphocyte and antithymocyte globulins. Transplantation 1991;51(3):669–73.

[44] Rebellato LM, Gross U, Verbanac KM, et al. A comprehensive definition of the major antibody specificities in polyclonal rabbit antithymocyte globulin. Transplantation 1994; 57(5):685–94.

[45] Bourdage JS, Hamlin DM. Comparative polyclonal antithymocyte globulin and antilymphocyte/antilymphoblast globulin anti-CD antigen analysis by flow cytometry. Transplantation 1995;59(8):1194–200.

[46] Kirk AD, Hale DA, Mannon RB, et al. Results from a human renal allograft tolerance trial evaluating the humanized CD52-specific monoclonal antibody alemtuzumab (CAMPATH-1H). Transplantation 2003;76(1):120–9.

[47] Simpson D. T-cell depleting antibodies: new hope for induction of allograft tolerance in bone marrow transplantation? BioDrugs 2003;17(3):147–54.

[48] Hale G, Hoang T, Prospero T, et al. Removal of T cells from bone marrow for transplantation. Comparison of rat monoclonal anti-lymphocyte antibodies of different isotypes. Mol Biol Med 1983;1(3):305–19.

[49] Hale G, Bright S, Chumbley G, et al. Removal of T cells from bone marrow for transplantation: a monoclonal antilymphocyte antibody that fixes human complement. Blood 1983; 62(4):873–82.

[50] Dyer MJ, Hale G, Hayhoe FG, et al. Effects of CAMPATH-1 antibodies in vivo in patients with lymphoid malignancies: influence of antibody isotype. Blood 1989;73(6):1431–9.

[51] Calne R, Friend P, Moffatt S, et al. Prope tolerance, perioperative campath 1H, and low-dose cyclosporin monotherapy in renal allograft recipients. Lancet 1998;351(9117): 1701–2.

[52] Prlic M, Jameson SC. Homeostatic expansion versus antigen-driven proliferation: common ends by different means? Microbes Infect 2002;4(5):531–7.

[53] Wu Z, Bensinger SJ, Zhang J, et al. Homeostatic proliferation is a barrier to transplantation tolerance. Nat Med 2004;10(1):87–92.

[54] Webster AC, Playford EG, Higgins G, et al. Interleukin 2 receptor antagonists for renal transplant recipients: a meta-analysis of randomized trials. Transplantation 2004;77(2): 166–76.

[55] Adu D, Cockwell P, Ives NJ, et al. Interleukin-2 receptor monoclonal antibodies in renal transplantation: meta-analysis of randomised trials. BMJ 2003;326(7393):789.

[56] Li XC, Roy-Chaudhury P, Hancock WW, et al. IL-2 and IL-4 double knockout mice reject islet allografts: a role for novel T cell growth factors in allograft rejection. J Immunol 1998; 161(2):890–6.

[57] Kircher B, Latzer K, Gastl G, et al. Comparative in vitro study of the immunomodulatory activity of humanized and chimeric anti-CD25 monoclonal antibodies. Clin Exp Immunol 2003;134(3):426–30.

[58] Bradley BA. The role of HLA matching in transplantation. Immunol Lett 1991;29(1–2): 55–9.

[59] Iwaki Y, Lau M, Cook DJ, et al. Crossmatching with B and T cells and flow cytometry. Clin Transpl 1986;1:277–84.

[60] Patel R, Terasaki PI. Significance of the positive crossmatch test in kidney transplantation. N Engl J Med 1969;280(14):735–9.

[61] Meier-Kriesche HU, Schold JD, Kaplan B. Long-term renal allograft survival: have we made significant progress or is it time to rethink our analytic and therapeutic strategies? Am J Transplant 2004;4(8):1289–95.

[62] Meier-Kriesche HU, Schold JD, Srinivas TR, et al. Lack of improvement in renal allograft survival despite a marked decrease in acute rejection rates over the most recent era. Am J Transplant 2004;4(3):378–83.

[63] Lenschow DJ, Zeng Y, Thistlethwaite JR, et al. Long-term survival of xenogeneic pancreatic islet grafts induced by CTLA4Ig. Science 1992;257(5071):789–92.

[64] Kirk AD, Harlan DM, Armstrong NN, et al. CTLA4-Ig and anti-CD40 ligand prevent renal allograft rejection in primates. Proc Natl Acad Sci U S A 1997;94(16):8789–94.

[65] Pearson TC, Trambley J, Odom K, et al. Anti-CD40 therapy extends renal allograft survival in rhesus macaques. Transplantation 2002;74(7):933–40.

[66] Vincenti F. Chronic induction. What's new in the pipeline. Contrib Nephrol 2005;146:22–9.

[67] Billingham RE, Brent L, Medawar PB. Actively acquired tolerance of foreign cells. Nature 1953;172(4379):603–6.

[68] Kawai T, Cosimi AB, Colvin RB, et al. Mixed allogeneic chimerism and renal allograft tolerance in cynomolgus monkeys. Transplantation 1995;59(2):256–62.

[69] Hamawi K, Magalhaes-Silverman M, Bertolatus JA. Outcomes of renal transplantation following bone marrow transplantation. Am J Transplant 2003;3(3):301–5.

[70] Buhler LH, Spitzer TR, Sykes M, et al. Induction of kidney allograft tolerance after transient lymphohematopoietic chimerism in patients with multiple myeloma and end-stage renal disease. Transplantation 2002;74(10):1405–9.

[71] Millan MT, Shizuru JA, Hoffmann P, et al. Mixed chimerism and immunosuppressive drug withdrawal after HLA-mismatched kidney and hematopoietic progenitor transplantation. Transplantation 2002;73(9):1386–91.

[72] Rao AS, Dvorchik I, Dodson F, et al. Donor bone marrow infusion in liver recipients: effect on the occurrence of acute cellular rejection. Transplant Proc 2001;33(1–2):1352.

[73] Shapiro R, Rao AS, Corry RJ, et al. Kidney transplantation with bone marrow augmentation: five-year outcomes. Transplant Proc 2001;33(1–2):1134–5.

[74] Pham SM, Rao AS, Zeevi A, et al. Effects of donor bone marrow infusion in clinical lung transplantation. Ann Thorac Surg 2000;69(2):345–50.

[75] Corry RJ, Chakrabarti PK, Shapiro R, et al. Simultaneous administration of adjuvant donor bone marrow in pancreas transplant recipients. Ann Surg 1999;230(3):372–9.

[76] Tryphonopoulos P, Tzakis AG, Weppler D, et al. The role of donor bone marrow infusions in withdrawal of immunosuppression in adult liver allotransplantation. Am J Transplant 2005;5(3):608–13.

[77] Contreras JL, Wang PX, Eckhoff DE, et al. Peritransplant tolerance induction with anti-CD3-immunotoxin: a matter of proinflammatory cytokine control. Transplantation 1998; 65(9):1159–69.

[78] Thomas JM, Neville DM, Contreras JL, et al. Preclinical studies of allograft tolerance in rhesus monkeys: a novel anti-CD3-immunotoxin given peritransplant with donor bone marrow induces operational tolerance to kidney allografts. Transplantation 1997;64(1):124–35.

[79] Thomas JM, Eckhoff DE, Contreras JL, et al. Durable donor-specific T and B cell tolerance in rhesus macaques induced with peritransplantation anti-CD3 immunotoxin and deoxyspergualin: absence of chronic allograft nephropathy. Transplantation 2000;69(12):2497–503.

[80] McCurry KR, Iacono A, Zeevi A, et al. Early outcomes in human lung transplantation with thymoglobulin or Campath-1H for recipient pretreatment followed by posttransplant tacrolimus near-monotherapy. J Thorac Cardiovasc Surg 2005;130(2):528–37.

[81] Watson CJ, Bradley JA, Friend PJ, et al. Alemtuzumab (CAMPATH 1H) induction therapy in cadaveric kidney transplantation–efficacy and safety at five years. Am J Transplant 2005; 5(6):1347–53.

SURGICAL
CLINICS OF
NORTH AMERICA

ELSEVIER
SAUNDERS

Surg Clin N Am 86 (2006) 1127–1145

# Infections Complicating Solid Organ Transplantation

## Staci A. Fischer, MD

*Brown Medical School, Division of Transplant Infectious Diseases, Rhode Island Hospital,*
*593 Eddy Street, Providence, RI 02903, USA*

In 2005, more than 28,000 solid organ transplants were performed in the United States [1]. Accompanying the life-saving organ transplant for each of these patients was the concomitant need for immunosuppression and a heightened risk of infection. Advances in immune suppression have resulted in improved allograft survival; nevertheless, the risk of infection with a myriad of organisms persists. In the past a timetable of infection following organ transplantation [2] helped guide diagnostic considerations when transplant recipients developed fever. Recent changes in immune suppression and the use of prophylactic antimicrobial agents have altered the classic timing of post-transplant infections. Clinicians must be aware of the changing scope of infections complicating transplantation and remain vigilant in the evaluation of potential infections following transplantation.

## Challenges to the clinician

Diagnosing infection in the transplant recipient can be difficult [3]. Corticosteroids commonly result in a lowering of core body temperature, so that infections might not produce a recognizable fever. Knowledge of the patient's baseline temperature (which might be 96–97° F) is important in evaluating new symptoms. In addition, azathioprine, mycophenolate, and prophylactic antimicrobials including valganciclovir and trimethoprim-sulfamethoxazole frequently cause leukopenia, so the solid organ recipient may have a low baseline leukocyte count. With infection, a relative leukocytosis can appear to be a normal leukocyte count without knowledge of the patient's baseline studies.

*E-mail address:* sfischer@lifespan.org

0039-6109/06/$ - see front matter © 2006 Elsevier Inc. All rights reserved.
doi:10.1016/j.suc.2006.06.005
*surgical.theclinics.com*

Certain tests used to commonly diagnose infection, such as serology and nuclear medicine studies, have a low sensitivity in this patient population. Infection with immunomodulating viruses such as cytomegalovirus (CMV) and Hepatitis C may further impact the risk, clinical presentation, and diagnosis of other opportunistic infections. Acute rejection can mimic infection, producing fever and other signs and symptoms suggestive of infection.

## Epidemiology of infection following solid organ transplantation

Infection can be transmitted by donor tissues or blood products, or acquired from the hospital environment or the home setting. Careful screening of potential solid organ transplant recipients for underlying infection, as well as education in the utility of common infection prevention methods (e.g., hand hygiene, certain vaccinations, safe food preparation and pet handling), may help prevent some infections in the post-transplant period [4–6]. Guidelines for the screening, monitoring, and reporting of infectious disease complications of organ transplantation have been published recently [7].

## Timing of post-transplant infections

Early experience with solid organ transplantation suggested that certain infections exhibited a temporal pattern following transplantation, creating a timeline [2,8]. Although changes in immunosuppression regimens and the use of prophylactic antimicrobials have altered that timeline, certain general principles remain accurate.

In the initial weeks following organ transplantation, infection can develop from several sources: incubating infection in the recipient, donor infection transmitted with the allograft, contamination during procurement and transport, or, most commonly, nosocomial infection following transplant surgery, including urinary tract infections (UTIs), pneumonia, intravenous catheter-related infections, and postoperative wound infections. Organisms reported to be transmitted with allografts are listed in Box 1. Infection with opportunistic pathogens such as CMV, *Aspergillus*, and *Legionella pneumophila* are distinctly uncommon in the first month following transplantation and generally present 1 to 6 months following transplantation. Some opportunists, notably *Cryptococcus neoformans*, usually cause infection more than 6 months following transplantation.

## Organ-specific considerations

Post-transplant anatomy, allograft ischemia, and local immunologic effects contribute to a higher risk of infection in the allograft itself. Renal

**Box 1. Donor-transmitted Infections**

| | |
|---|---|
| Bacterial | Enteric Gram-negative bacilli |
| | *Pseudomonas aeruginosa* |
| | *Staphylococcus aureus* (including methicillin-resistant *S aureus* [MRSA]) |
| | *Bacteroides fragilis* |
| | *Treponema pallidum* (syphilis) |
| | *Salmonella* spp |
| | *Stenotrophomonas maltophilia* |
| | *Streptococcus milleri* |
| | |
| Viral | Cytomegalovirus (CMV) |
| | Epstein-Barr virus (EBV) |
| | Herpes simplex virus |
| | Hepatitis B, C, and delta hepatitis |
| | HIV |
| | Adenovirus |
| | Rabies virus |
| | West Nile virus |
| | Parvovirus B19 |
| | Polyoma virus (BK, JC) |
| | Lymphocytic chorimeningitis virus |
| | |
| Fungal | *Candida* spp |
| | *Histoplasma capsulatum* |
| | *Cryptococcus neoformans* |
| | *Aspergillus fumigatus* |
| | *Coccidioides immitus* |
| | Pneumocystis jiroveci |
| | |
| Protozoal | *Toxoplasma gondii* |
| | *Strongyloides stercoralis* |
| | *Trypanosoma cruzi* |
| | *Babesia microti* |
| | *Leishmania donovanii* |
| | *Plasmodium* spp (malaria) |
| | |
| Mycobacterial | *Mycobacterium tuberculosis* |
| | *Mycobacterium chelonae* |
| | |
| Prion disease | Creutzfeld-Jakob agent |

transplant recipients are at life-long risk of pyelonephritis caused, in part, by the shorter length and more acute angle of the transplanted ureter relative to native anatomy, the high incidence of reflux, and ischemic and immunologic injury to the allograft [9,10]. Bacteremia complicating urinary tract infection is often caused by concomitant transplant pyelonephritis and should be treated with a longer course of antibiotics (at least 14 days) in the kidney transplant recipient. Pain overlying the allograft should raise suspicion for pyelonephritis and acute rejection.

BK virus is a human polyoma virus that has particular significance in the renal transplant population. Symptomatic infection is relatively unique to this population and can mimic acute rejection clinically and pathologically [11]. BK nephropathy results in significant permanent renal dysfunction in most cases and carries a 50% or greater risk of allograft loss [12]. Up to 80% of adults have serologic evidence of prior infection with this polyoma virus, which remains latent in renal epithelial cells [9]. Reactivation of infection from donor or recipient tissue can occur following renal transplantation, resulting in declining allograft function, interstitial nephritis resembling acute rejection, ureteral stenosis, or hemorrhagic cystitis [13,14]. Diagnosis is made by renal biopsy with immunohistochemical staining, although urine cytology to identify "decoy cells" and polymerase chain reaction (PCR) testing of blood for viral DNA may be helpful [15,16]. The first line of treatment consists of decreasing immunosuppression. Leflunomide and low-dose cidofovir have been reported to be of benefit in patients who have persistent infection and renal dysfunction [16,17].

Liver transplantation is frequently complicated by infection. This patient population is at increased risk of infection as a result of underlying neutrophil dysfunction, intensive care unit hospitalization and frequent exposure to broad-spectrum antimicrobials prior to transplantation [18–20]. In the initial weeks after transplantation, wound infection, anastomotic leak with intra-abdominal abscess formation, and bacteremia with enteric organisms such as *Enterobacter* species, *Escherichia coli*, *Klebsiella pneumoniae*, *Pseudomonas aeruginosa, and Enterococcus* (including vancomycin-resistant *Enterococcus*) occur [21]. Percutaneous T-tubes placed to protect the biliary anastomosis predispose to bacteremia and cholangitis with cutaneous flora, including staphylococci, increasingly methicillin-resistant *Staphylococcus* (MRSA) [22]. Operative factors, including duration of surgery ($\geq 8$ hours) and intra-operative blood transfusion requirements ($> 2$ blood volumes), have been predictive of early postoperative infection [21]. Postoperative thrombosis, hematoma, or anastomotic leaks predispose to bacterial and candidal infection. Hepatic abscess in this population can complicate hepatic artery thrombosis or cholangitis and can be polymicrobial, involving the Enterobacteriaceae, *Streptococcus milleri*, and *Bacteroides fragilis* [23]. Bacteremia is common in this setting, and culture of abscess contents for organism identification and susceptibility testing is recommended. Infections can be polymicrobial, and increasing antimicrobial resistance has been noted in this patient population [24,25].

Candida infections occur in up to 35% of liver transplant recipients and are associated with a mortality rate of 23% to 60% [26,27]. Overgrowth of Candida in the gut can result in translocation with intra-abdominal infection and hematogenous dissemination. Prophylactic antifungal agents such as fluconazole and itraconazole are effective in reducing the incidence of invasive Candida infections following liver transplantation, but they have contributed to growing resistance in yeasts [28]. The liver transplant recipient with bile duct obstruction or vascular complications such as portal vein or hepatic artery thrombosis can develop multiple hepatic abscesses and recurrent polymicrobial bloodstream infection. Unexplained fever or bacteremia in the first few weeks after liver transplantation should raise suspicion of an underlying vascular complication.

Pancreas transplantation can be complicated by intra-abdominal infections as a result of duodenal anastomotic leaks, resulting in fever, nausea, vomiting, and abdominal pain and may result in allograft loss [29,30]. Ultrasound or CT may reveal a peri-pancreatic fluid collection, which can be difficult to interpret in the early postoperative period. Peri-pancreatic abscesses are most commonly caused by enteric bacteria, including E coli, Klebsiella, Enterococcus, and Candida species and can be polymicrobial. Drainage (for culture) and repair of any anastomotic leaks are critical to resolution. Repeat laparotomy for intra-abdominal infection is associated with a 60% or higher risk of graft loss [31]. Bladder-drained pancreas transplantation is associated with a higher risk of UTIs and wound infection with Candida [32]. Although glycemic control is no longer an issue after successful pancreas transplantation, recipients remain at life-long risk for infectious complications of long-standing microvascular disease and peripheral neuropathy, including foot ulcerations and consequent osteomyelitis.

Cardiac transplant recipients are at high risk for pneumonia caused by bacteria (including Legionella, discussed below) and fungi, including Aspergillus and Pneumocystis jiroveci [33–38]. Sternal wound infection and mediastinitis can develop, most commonly involving staphylococci or Gram-negative bacilli. Patients present in the first few weeks following transplantation with fever and chest discomfort, and they frequently require surgical debridement and prolonged antimicrobial courses [39,40]. Heart transplant recipients are at particular risk for infection with Toxoplasma gondii, a protozoan that can be transmitted with the allograft because of its latency in cardiac muscle [41]. The seronegative recipient of a seropositive heart can develop myocarditis mimicking acute rejection, with tachyzoites or cysts with myocyte necrosis visualized in endomyocardial biopsies, and disseminated infection can occur. Symptoms typically begin 4 to 6 weeks after transplantation [41]. Reactivation of latent infection can occur in all solid organ transplant recipients, causing encephalitis.

Lung transplantation is frequently complicated by pneumonia acquired from pretransplant airway colonization of the donor or recipient or from the community or hospital setting. Pre-transplant airway colonization with resistant organisms including *P aeruginosa*, atypical mycobacteria, and *Burkholderia cepacia* can pose significant risk of allograft infection and sepsis; for many centers, colonization with the latter is an absolute contraindication to transplantation [42]. Because the allograft itself is constantly exposed to the environment, prevention of infection is difficult and common viruses (eg, adenovirus, respiratory syncytial virus, influenza, metapneumovirus, parainfluenza virus) can cause severe disease, sometimes years after successful lung transplantation [43–45].

Pneumonia caused by ubiquitous molds including *Aspergillus* is common following lung transplantation, particularly after single-lung transplantation [42]. Patients present with dyspnea, often accompanied by fever and malaise; productive cough and hemoptysis might be absent. Infection of the bronchial anastomosis with tracheobronchitis can occur, in which chest radiographs might be unremarkable, or focal consolidations with cavitation can be seen with invasive pulmonary aspergillosis. Disseminated disease carries a mortality rate of 35% [42]. Because of the morbidity and mortality associated with mold infection, prophylaxis with agents such as inhaled amphotericin B, itraconazole, or voriconazole is commonplace in this patient group [46]. Differentiation of colonization and invasive infection with this ubiquitous mold is critical in evaluating the lung transplant recipient who has suspected pulmonary infection, and transbronchial biopsy to look for tissue invasion is important.

Because of the plethora of organisms of potential harm to lung transplant recipients and the availability of newer antiviral, antibacterial, and antifungal agents to treat infections, rapid diagnostic procedures including bronchoscopy with bronchoalveolar lavage for cultures are critical for diagnosis and appropriate treatment in the lung transplant recipient with pneumonia.

## Opportunistic pathogens of importance in solid organ transplantation

### Cytomegalovirus (CMV)

CMV is the most important viral pathogen affecting transplant recipients [8,47,48]. Although infection has traditionally occurred 1 to 3 months following transplantation, patients who have a history of acute allograft rejection, particularly those treated with antilymphocyte therapies, can develop CMV infection and disease later in the post-transplant course. Even in patients who have not had aggressive anti-rejection treatment, late-onset disease is increasingly seen [49], so that CMV should be considered in the differential diagnosis in many solid organ transplant recipients who present with fever. In addition, many programs recommend prolonged administration of CMV prophylaxis (beyond 3 months), especially for CMV-seronegative recipients of CMV-seropositive allografts. This may delay CMV infection until after the period after prophylaxis, when immune function is better constituted.

Eighty to 90% of adults are CMV-seropositive (anti-CMV IgG-positive). Primary infection usually occurs in childhood or adolescence and can be asymptomatic or present with a nonspecific febrile illness or heterophile-negative mononucleosis syndrome. Latent infection is maintained in endothelial cells, hematopoietic cells, peripheral lymphocytes, and monocytes [47], from which infection can reactivate with immunosuppression. Transplant recipients can also acquire CMV infection from the allograft itself, from blood products, or by way of natural infection, and superinfections can occur. Recipients at highest risk of infection and serious disease are those who were seronegative pretransplant (R–) and received an allograft from a seropositive donor (D+).

CMV in the transplant recipient can be asymptomatic or may cause a febrile illness without end-organ involvement, commonly referred to as "CMV syndrome." These patients have fever, often with myalgias, anorexia, and fatigue. Leukopenia, thrombocytopenia and mildly elevated transaminases can be seen. On occasion, the patients develop thrombocytopenia and mildly elevated transaminases. Atypical lymphocytosis (5–10% of lymphocytes) and lymphadenopathy may be seen. In some cases, prolonged fever is the only symptom present.

CMV can also cause invasive disease, often affecting the allograft itself (eg, pancreatitis in the pancreas recipient, hepatitis in the liver recipient), simulating rejection clinically and diagnosed by allograft biopsy. CMV pneumonitis is common following lung transplantation, in part because of the implantation of an organ rich in lymphatic tissue latently infected with CMV in seropositive donors [48]. Co-infection with other pathogens, including viruses and *Pneumocystis* (discussed below) can occur, often resulting in more severe disease. Because CMV is associated with vascular injury and chronic allograft injury or bronchiolitis obliterans syndrome, prevention of CMV infection is particularly important in the lung transplant population [50].

Outside of the allograft, CMV disease most commonly manifests as infection in the gastrointestinal tract following solid organ transplantation. Ulcerative lesions can develop anywhere from the mouth to the anus, presenting with diarrhea, bleeding, nausea, bloating, emesis, dyspepsia, or dysphagia. Mass lesions of the gastrointestinal tract can be seen, mimicking lymphoma or other malignancies. CMV pneumonitis carries a significant mortality rate, particularly in lung and heart–lung transplant recipients, who are at highest risk [48]. Patients present with fever, dyspnea, and a non-productive cough and usually have bilateral interstitial infiltrates on chest radiographs. CMV hepatitis, while most common in liver transplant recipients, can occur in any organ recipient, presenting with fever and elevated transaminases and alkaline phosphatase. Other manifestations of

CMV disease include pancreatitis (most common in pancreas recipients), encephalitis, transverse myelitis, endometritis, cutaneous ulcerations, and epididymitis [47]. CMV retinitis, a manifestation common in patients with advanced HIV infection, is distinctly unusual in solid organ transplant recipients and presents substantially later than other sites of CMV disease [50,51].

CMV is important not only for the direct effect of infection on tissues (including the allograft itself) but also for its immunomodulatory effects, which can predispose patients to other infections and enhance allorecognition. A number of bacterial and fungal infections have been reported to complicate CMV in solid organ transplantation [52–54]. The association of CMV with chronic rejection in solid organ transplant recipients, while incompletely explained to date, makes prevention, early diagnosis, and effective treatment of this common post-transplant infection critical.

A number of strategies have been studied to prevent CMV infection following transplantation, including the use of prophylactic ganciclovir (intravenously or orally), valganciclovir, or immune globulin therapy in all patients at risk of CMV [55–60]. Some centers follow a preemptive strategy, monitoring all recipients at risk with sensitive, quantitative viral diagnostic tests including PCR and pp65 antigenemia; this approach exposes only those patients who have evidence of replicating virus to antiviral agents and their toxicities, but it requires frequent patient monitoring [61–63]. It is more common for centers to recommend CMV prophylaxis to for a defined period after transplantation (usually 3-6 months).

Diagnosis of CMV infection is best made by histologic examination of involved tissue—which reveals the presence of characteristic intracellular inclusions—with immunohistochemical confirmation. Other diagnostic techniques include viral culture (including shell-vial cultures), antigenemia assays, and PCR [47]. Each of these must be evaluated in the appropriate clinical setting because asymptomatic shedding of CMV occurs frequently and must be differentiated from invasive disease. Ganciclovir and valganciclovir are the mainstays of treatment of CMV infection and disease, although ganciclovir resistance has been reported in the solid organ transplant setting [64,65].

### *Aspergillus* and other molds

Although *Candida* species are the most common fungal pathogens infecting solid organ transplant recipients, molds such as *Aspergillus* remain an important cause of morbidity and mortality. Although uncommon following renal transplantation, invasive aspergillosis has been reported in up to 8% of liver transplant recipients and in up to 15% of heart and lung transplant recipients [66]. *Aspergillus* is ubiquitous in the environment and has caused outbreaks of infection in transplant units during hospital construction [67]. Tracheobronchitis, pneumonia, brain abscesses, and cutaneous, urinary, and disseminated disease have been reported and present within the first 6 months following transplantation in most cases. Cultures of respiratory secretions lack sensitivity and specificity for the diagnosis of aspergillosis; histopathologic examination and culture of tissue specimens obtained by biopsy are key diagnostic studies. Although amphotericin B is the gold standard for antifungal therapy, newer agents such as voriconazole might be even more efficacious [68]. The mortality rate of *Aspergillus* infection remains greater than 50% in this patient population, so prophylaxis against this pathogen is nearly universal in the highest-risk population (ie, patients undergoing lung transplantation) [69]. Many other molds, which possess varying antifungal susceptibilities, are capable of causing invasive infection following solid organ transplantation, so that culture of biopsied tissue specimens is crucial [70].

### Pneumocystis jiroveci

*P jiroveci* (previously known as *Pneumocystis carinii*) is a fungus that causes life-threatening pneumonia in immunocompromised hosts, including solid organ transplant recipients. Those undergoing lung and heart–lung transplantation are at greatest risk [71]. Patients typically present 2 to 12 months after transplantation with fever, nonproductive cough, and dyspnea [22,72]. Bilateral interstitial infiltrates are seen on chest radiographs, with rapid progression noted over days to weeks if untreated. Extrapulmonary disease including involvement of the liver, spleen, lymph nodes, and bone marrow has been described [73]. Because the organism is difficult to culture, diagnosis is made by histopathologic demonstration of the organism in infected tissue or bronchoalveolar lavage fluid, frequently using direct fluorescent antibody staining specific to the organism. Although non-invasive techniques such as induced sputum are often adequate for diagnosis of *Pneumocystis* pneumonia in HIV-infected patients, the organism burden in the transplant recipient is significantly lower, so that bronchoscopy is often needed to make a diagnosis. Co-infection with other respiratory opportunistic pathogens such as CMV can occur [22]. Treatment with trimethoprim–sulfamethoxazole is effective in most cases, and this agent is used for prophylaxis against infection for at least 12 months following transplantation in most centers [74,75].

### Legionella pneumophila

*Legionella* remains an important opportunistic pathogen in the solid organ transplant population. Infection is acquired via inhalation of aerosols or microaspiration of water contaminated with the organism [76]. Nosocomial outbreaks of legionellosis have been described in transplant centers, although community-acquired infection also occurs [77,78]. Infection can occur at any time following transplantation, but it is most common 2 to 6 months after transplant or following augmented immunosuppression for acute rejection [76,77]. Symptoms of infection include fever, minimally productive cough, and dyspnea associated with myalgias, anorexia, headache, and diarrhea in some cases; hyponatremia and relative bradycardia may also be present. Chest radiographs reveal multi-focal alveolar infiltrates, with nodular, cavitating infiltrates seen in some patients. Acute renal failure is common in this setting, and pleural effusions, empyema, and lung abscesses can develop [79,80]. Diagnosis can be made by urine *Legionella* antigen testing, which detects the major *L pneumophila* serogroup seen in the United States, or by way of direct fluorescent antibody (DFA) staining or specialized culture of respiratory secretions or lung tissue specimens [81]. *Legionella micdadei* has also been reported to cause pneumonia in renal and liver transplant recipients. It can be diagnosed by DFA or immunohistochemical staining of lung tissue [82]. Treatment of legionellosis includes fluoroquinolones (eg, ciprofloxacin and levofloxacin) and macrolides (eg, azithromycin and clarithromycin), although the latter have significant drug interactions with calcineurin inhibitors and sirolimus and must be used with caution in the post-transplant population (see Table 1). Patients should receive a 21-day course of therapy for *Legionella* pneumonia.

### *Toxoplasma gondii*

*T gondii* is a coccidian parasite of cats that is acquired by ingestion of oocysts in raw vegetables or undercooked meat products. It can be transmitted by way of the allograft itself in cardiac transplant recipients. Although primary infection is often asymptomatic, latent infection in the CNS, eye, bone, smooth muscle, and cardiac muscle can reactivate with immune suppression. The incidence of toxoplasmosis is highest in heart and heart–lung transplant recipients, in whom donor-transmitted disease can present with disseminated infection in the first 2 weeks following transplantation [41]. Primary and reactivation disease is seen in all organ transplant groups and may present with lymphadenopathy, mononucleosis-like illness, myocarditis, pneumonitis, fulminant hepatitis, encephalitis, chorioretinitis, or disseminated disease, usually in the first 3 months following organ transplantation [83–85]. With routine trimethoprim–sulfamethoxazole prophylaxis following transplantation, toxoplasmosis is less frequent than previously described, although late onset disease can be seen, particularly involving the CNS [86–88]. Diagnosis can be made by periodic acid-Schiff staining of tissue specimens or PCR testing of bronchoalveolar lavage fluid. Cerebrospinal fluid and serology may be useful in some cases. The mortality rate of *Toxoplasma* infection in transplant recipients is 65% to 100%, so that early diagnosis is critical [84].

Table 1
Antimicrobial drug interactions with immunosuppressive agents [101–103]

| Antimicrobial agent | Cyclosporine | Tacrolimus | Sirolimus |
| --- | --- | --- | --- |
| Ciprofloxacin | ⇑ levels | | |
| Ofloxacin | ⇑ levels | | |
| Levofloxacin | No effect | No effect | No effect |
| Gatifloxacin | No effect | No effect | No effect |
| Moxifloxacin | No effect | No effect | No effect |
| Nalidixic acid | ⇑ levels | | |
| Erythromycin | ⇑ levels | ⇑ levels | ⇑ levels |
| Clarithromycin | ⇑ levels | ⇑ levels | ⇑ levels |
| Azithromycin | ⇑ levels | | |
| Telithromycin | ⇑ levels | ⇑ levels | ⇑ levels |
| Nafcillin | ⇓ levels | | |
| Clindamycin | ⇓ levels | | |
| Imipenem/cilastatin | ⇑ levels | | |
| Chloramphenicol | | ⇑ levels | |
| Quinupristin/dalfopristin | ⇑ levels | ⇑ levels | |
| Metronidazole | ⇑ levels | ⇑ levels | |
| Rifampin | ⇓ levels | ⇓ levels | ⇓ levels |
| Rifabutin | ⇓ levels | ⇓ levels | ⇓ levels |
| Dapsone | | ⇑ levels | |
| Sulfadiazine | ⇓ levels | | |
| Pyrazinamide | ⇓ levels | | |
| Caspofungin | * | ⇓ levels | |
| Micafungin | | | ⇑ levels |
| Fluconazole | ⇑ levels | ⇑ levels | ⇑ levels |
| Ketoconazole | ⇑ levels | ⇑ levels | ⇑ levels |
| Itraconaozle | ⇑ levels | ⇑ levels | Contraindicated |
| Voriconazole | ⇑ levels | ⇑ levels | Contraindicated |

* Cyclosporine increases serum levels of caspofungin and enhances the hepatotoxicity of this agent.

## *Cryptococcus neoformans*

*C neoformans* is an encapsulated yeast found in soil and avian guano. It has been reported to cause pneumonia, meningitis, cellulitis, prostatitis, osteomyelitis, and disseminated infection following solid organ transplantation [89,90]. Patients acquire infection by way of inhalation of airborne fungi from ubiquitous environmental sources. Certain birds, including pigeons and cockatoos, have been associated with infection in the transplant setting [91]. Infection often occurs more than 1 year after transplantation and presents with headache, confusion, and lethargy in those who have CNS disease or with alveolar, nodular, or cavitary infiltrates in those who have pneumonia, with pleural effusions in some cases [92,93]. Meningismus is rarely present, but cerebrospinal fluid reveals encapsulated yeast on India ink testing or cryptococcal antigen testing. Increasingly, cutaneous and osteoarticular disease has been reported in solid organ transplant recipients, in which biopsies and culture demonstrate the organism [94–96]. Treatment consists of fluconazole or amphotericin B for at least 6 weeks.

## Listeria monocytogenes

*L monocytogenes* is a cause of bacteremia and meningitis following solid organ transplantation. Infection has been reported to occur within the first month post-transplant, but it more commonly develops months to years after transplantation [97]. Although meningitis and bacteremia are most commonly reported, endocarditis, endophthalmitis, brain abscess, and allograft involvement (hepatitis in liver transplant recipients and myocarditis in heart transplant recipients) have been described [98–100]. In *Listeria* meningitis, Gram stains of cerebrospinal fluid demonstrate the characteristic Gram-positive bacilli in only 40% of patients; culture is diagnostic. *Listeria* is inherently resistant to the third-generation cephalosporins commonly used in the empiric treatment of bacterial meningitis. Ampicillin is the drug of choice for treatment of listeriosis and should be administered for 21 days; trimethoprim–sulfamethoxazole may be substituted in penicillin-allergic patients.

## Approach to the solid organ transplant patient with fever

In evaluating the transplant recipient with fever, the timing of presentation post-transplant and organ-specific infections should be considered. The infectious disease work-up differs based on the organ transplanted, the interval from transplantation, and local epidemiologic phenomena. Recent exposure to high doses of immunosuppression, particularly corticosteroid boluses or antilymphocyte preparations used in the treatment of rejection, dramatically increase the risk of infection compared with maintenance doses of immunosuppressive drugs. Transplant recipients, like other immunocompromised hosts, are classically referred to as "sentinel chickens" because they are the first in the hospital or community setting to develop infection with new and emerging pathogens, bringing local outbreaks to light. They can acquire food-borne pathogens with ingestion of contaminated raw fruits and vegetables or undercooked meat (poultry or pork) and are at risk of more severe manifestations of such infections, best exemplified by the higher incidence of bacteremia complicating *Salmonella* infections in this population. Travel to domestic and foreign destinations can predispose the transplant recipient to infection with food-borne, arthropod-borne, and tick-borne infections as well as to infection with endemic fungi such as *Coccidioides immitus* or *Histoplasma capsulatum*. Such infections might be self-limited in the immunocompetent host (often the patient's travel partner), but infection can become disseminated and may be fatal in the transplant patient. As a result, the diagnostic

Table 2
Approach to the diagnosis of infection in the solid organ transplant recipient with fever

| Syndrome | Recommended initial diagnostic evaluation* |
| --- | --- |
| Fever without localizing findings | Urinalysis and urine culture<br>Chest radiograph<br>Blood cultures<br>CMV PCR<br>PPD and anergy profile |
| Pulmonary infiltrates<br>Alveolar | PPD and anergy profile<br>Blood cultures<br>Sputum Gram stain and culture<br>Urine *Legionella* antigen<br>Sputum AFB smear and culture<br>Sputum fungal smear and culture<br>Urine *Histoplasma* antigen in endemic areas<br>Bronchoscopy if fever and infiltrates persist |
| Interstitial | Above workup plus CMV PCR<br>Urine *Histoplasma* antigen or *Cocciodioides* serology in endemic areas<br>Bronchoscopy with transbronchial biopsy if fever and infiltrates persist<br>Bronchoalveolar lavage fluid should be submitted for bacterial, viral, AFB, and fungal cultures; DFA and culture for *Legionella*; DFA for *Pneumocystis jiroveci*; CMV PCR; cytology; modified AFB smear and culture (to look for *Nocardia*). |
| CNS symptoms | MRI brain with gadolinium<br>Lumbar puncture with cell count and differential; bacterial, AFB, viral and fungal cultures, cryptococcal antigen, cytology.<br>Consider CMV, EBV, West Nile virus, and arbovirus testing (PCR and/or serology) based on epidemiology, timing post-transplant and local patterns of infection.<br>Biopsy of mass lesions and/or meninges if above work-up is unrevealing and symptoms and signs of infection persist. |
| Diarrhea | Stool cultures (for *Salmonella*, *Shigella*, *Campylobacter*)<br>Stool for *Clostridium difficile* toxin testing<br>Stool for ova and parasites ($\times$3)<br>CMV PCR (on blood)<br>If stool studies are unrevealing and diarrhea persists, endoscopic evaluation with flexible sigmoidoscopy or colonosopy (with mucosal biopsy) is indicated. Immunohistochemical staining for CMV should be performed. |
| Lymphadenopathy | EBV PCR, CMV PCR (blood)<br>*Bartonella* (cat-scratch disease) serology<br>*Toxoplasma gondii* serology<br>PPD and anergy profile |

(*continued on next page*)

Table 2 (*continued*)

| Syndrome | Recommended initial diagnostic evaluation* |
|---|---|
| | Biopsy of involved lymph node is often diagnostic and should be performed quickly in this population to rule out post-transplant lymphoproliferative disorder and occult infections including tuberculosis. Node tissue should be submitted for histologic examination to look for atypical cells, granulomata, and cultures (aerobic, anaerobic, AFB, fungal and modified AFB). CT scan of the neck, chest, abdomen and pelvis might be useful to demonstrate the extent of nodal involvement. |

*Abbreviations:* Acid-fast bacillus, AFB; Direct fluorescent antigen testing, DFA; Purified protein derivative (tuberculin skin testing), PPD.

* Recommendations based on published data and clinical experience. Consultation with infectious disease specialists is recommended in patients in whom a source of fever cannot be identified after initial diagnostic evaluation.

evaluation of fever in this patient population should be detailed and complete, so that a microbiologic diagnosis can be made and appropriate antimicrobial therapy initiated.

Obtaining a detailed clinical and epidemiologic history helps guide the diagnostic work-up in the transplant recipient with fever; there is no one diagnostic algorithm such as the commonly utilized "pan-culture" approach to the post-operative patient who has fever. In many cases nonstandard cultures, molecular diagnostic testing, or tissue biopsy might be necessary to make a microbiologic diagnosis. Consultation with infectious disease specialists, especially those who have expertise in transplant infectious diseases, can be very helpful. Suggestions for the initial diagnostic evaluation of fever in the solid organ transplant recipient are listed in Table 2.

When an exhaustive evaluation for infection is unrevealing, consideration should be given to non-infectious causes of fever in this population, which include post-transplant lymphoproliferative disorder, allograft rejection, drug fever, and immunosuppressant-induced tissue damage (eg, sirolimus-induced pulmonary fibrosis and tacrolimus-induced CNS toxicity).

As graft and patient survival continue to improve following solid organ transplantation, a larger number of patients in the community are chronically immunosuppressed and at risk for infection. Prophylactic antimicrobials, such as those commonly given to prevent CMV, certain fungal infections, and *P jiroveci* are effective; however, the timing and clinical presentation of opportunistic pathogens, as well as the myriad of pathogens involved, is continually changing. Vigilance in the diagnostic evaluation of suspected infection in the solid organ transplant recipient will improve outcomes and quality of life following these life-saving procedures. Prompt diagnosis along with appropriate choice and duration of treatment of infectious diseases are essential in these challenging patients.

# References

[1] Organ Procurement and Transplantation Network. United Network for Organ Sharing, 2005. Available at: www.optn.org/latestdata/rptdata.asp. Accessed March 17, 2006.

[2] Rubin RH, Wolfson JS, Cosimi AB, et al. Infection in the renal transplant recipient. Am J Med 1981;70(2):405–11.

[3] Fischer SA, Trenholme GM, Levin S. Fever in the solid organ transplant patient. Infect Dis Clin N Am 1996;10(1):167–84.

[4] Patel R, Paya CV. Infections in solid-organ transplant recipients. Clin Microbiol Rev 1997; 10(1):86–124.

[5] Avery RK. Recipient screening prior to solid-organ transplantation. Clin Infect Dis 2002; 35:1513–9.

[6] Angulo FJ, Glaser CA, Juranek DD, et al. Caring for pets of immunocompromised persons. JAVMA 1994;205(12):1711–8.

[7] Humar A, Michaels M. American Society of Transplantation recommendations for screening, monitoring and reporting of infectious complications in immunosuppression trials in recipients of organ transplantation. Am J Transplant 2006;6:262–74.

[8] Fishman JA, Rubin RH. Infection in organ-transplant recipients. N Engl J Med 1998; 338(24):1741–51.

[9] Hibberd PL, Rubin RH. Renal transplantation and related infections. Sem Respir Infect 1993;8(3):216–24.

[10] Martinez-Marcos F, Cisneros J, Gentil M, et al. Prospective study of renal transplant infections in 50 consecutive patients. Eur J Clin Microbiol Infect Dis 1994;13(12):1023–8.

[11] Mylonakis E, Goes N, Rubin RH, et al. BK virus in solid organ transplant recipients: an emerging syndrome. Transplantation 2001;72:1587–92.

[12] Trofe J, Gaber LW, Stratta RJ, et al. Polyomavirus in kidney and kidney-pancreas transplant recipients. Transpl Infect Dis 2003;5:21–8.

[13] Nickeleit V, Hirsch HH, Binet IF, et al. Polyomavirus infection of renal allograft recipients: from latent infection to manifest disease. J Am Soc Nephrol 1999;10(5):1080–9.

[14] Ramos E, Drachenberg CB, Papdimitriou JC, et al. Clinical course of polyoma virus nephropathy in 67 renal transplant patients. J Am Soc Nephrol 2002;13(8):2145–51.

[15] Nickeleit V, Klimkait T, Binet IF, et al. Testing for polyomavirus type BK DNA in plasma to identify renal-allograft recipients with viral nephropathy. N Engl J Med 2000;342(18): 1309–62.

[16] Nickeleit V, Singh H, Mihatsch M. Polyomavirus nephropathy: morphology, pathophysiology, and clinical management. Curr Opin Nephr Hypertens 2003;12:599–605.

[17] Kadambi PV, Josephson MA, Williams J, et al. Treatment of refractory BK virus-associated nephropathy with cidofovir. Am J Transplant 2003;3:186–91.

[18] Winston DJ, Emmanouilides C, Busuttil RW. Infections in liver transplant recipients. Clin Infect Dis 1995;21:1077–91.

[19] Singh N. The current management of infectious diseases in the liver transplant recipient. Clin Liver Dis 2000;4(3):657–73.

[20] Paya CV, Hermans PE, Washington JA II, et al. Incidence, distribution, and outcome of episodes of infection in 100 orthotopic liver transplantations. Mayo Clin Proc 1989;64:555–64.

[21] George DL, Arnow PM, Fox AS, et al. Bacterial infection as a complication of liver transplantation: epidemiology and risk factors. Rev Infect Dis 1991;13:387–96.

[22] Kusne S, Dummer JS, Singh N, et al. Infections after liver transplantation: an analysis of 101 consecutive cases. Medicine 1988;67(2):132–43.

[23] Tachopoulou OA, Vogt DP, Henderson JM, et al. Hepatic abscess after liver transplantation: 1990–2000. Transplantation 2003;75(1):79–83.

[24] Singh N, Gayowsky T, Rihs JD, et al. Evolving trends in multiple-antibiotic-resistant bacteria in liver transplant recipients: a longitudinal study of antimicrobial susceptibility patterns. Liver Transpl 2001;7(1):22–6.

[25] Rubin RH. The direct and indirect effects of infection in liver transplantation: pathogenesis, impact, and clinical management. Curr Clin Top Infect Dis 2002;22:125–54.

[26] Wajszczuk CP, Dummer JS, Ho M, et al. Fungal infections in liver transplant recipients. Transplantation 1985;40(4):347–53.

[27] Husain S, Tollemar J, Dominguez EA, et al. Changes in the spectrum and risk factors for invasive Candidiasis in liver transplant recipients: prospective, multicenter, case-controlled study. Transplantation 2003;75(12):2023–9.

[28] Winston D, Pakrasi A, Busuttil RW. Prophylactic fluconazole in liver transplant recipients: a randomized, double-blind, placebo-controlled trial. Ann Intern Med 1999;121:729–37.

[29] Lumbreras C, Fernandez I, Velosa J, et al. Infectious complications following pancreatic transplantation: incidence, microbiological and clinical characteristics, and outcome. Clin Infect Dis 1995;20:514–20.

[30] Bassetti M, Salvalaggio PRO, Topal J, et al. Incidence, timing and site of infections among pancreas transplant recipients. J Hosp Infect 2004;56:184–90.

[31] Reddy KS, Stratta RJ, Shokouh-Amiri MH, et al. Surgical complications after pancreas transplantation with portal-enteric drainage. J Am Coll Surg 1999;89(3):305–13.

[32] Pirsch JD, Odorico JS, D'Alessandra AM, et al. Posttransplant infection in enteric versus bladder-drained simultaneous pancreas-kidney transplant recipients. Transplantation 1998;66(12):1746–50.

[33] Cisneros JM, Munoz P, Torre-Cisneros J, et al. Pneumonia after heart transplantation: a multiinstitutional study. Clin Infect Dis 1998;27:324–31.

[34] Schulman LL, Smith CR, Drusin R, et al. Respiratory complications of cardiac transplantation. Am J Med Sci 1988;296(1):1–10.

[35] Miller LW, Naftel DC, Bourge RC, et al. Infection after heart transplantation: a multiinstitutional study. J Heart Lung Transplant 1994;13(3):381–93.

[36] Montoya JG, Giraldo LF, Efron B, et al. Infectious complications among 620 consecutive heart transplant patients at Stanford University Medical Center. Clin Infect Dis 2001;33: 629–40.

[37] Petri WA Jr. Infections in heart transplant recipients. Clin Infect Dis 1994;18:141–8.

[38] Smart FW, Naftel DC, Costanza MR, et al. Risk factors for early, cumulative, and fatal infections after heart transplantation: a multiinstitutional study. J Heart Lung Transplant 1996;15(4):329–41.

[39] Anthuber M, Kemkes BM, Kreuzer E, et al. Mediastinitis and mycotic aneurysm of the aorta after orthotopic heart transplantation. Tex Heart Inst J 1991;18(3):186–93.

[40] Baldwin RT, Radovancevic B, Sweeney MS, et al. Bacterial mediastinitis after heart transplantation. J Heart Lung Transplant 1992;11(3):545–9.

[41] Luft BJ, Naot Y, Araujo FG, et al. Primary and reactivated *Toxoplasma* infection in patients with cardiac transplants. Ann Intern Med 1983;99:27–31.

[42] Westney GE, Kesten S, de Hoyos A, et al. *Aspergillus* infection in single and double lung transplant recipients. Transplantation 1996;61(6):915–9.

[43] Vilchez RA, McCurry K, Dauber J, et al. The epidemiology of parainfluenza virus infection in lung transplant recipients. Clin Infect Dis 2001;33:2004–8.

[44] Vilchez R, McCurry K, Dauber J, et al. Influenza and parainfluenza respiratory viral infection requiring admission in adult lung transplant recipients. Transplantation 2002;73(7): 1075–8.

[45] Ison MG, Hayden FG. Viral infections in immunocompromised patients: what's new with respiratory viruses? Curr Opin Infect Dis 2002;15:355–67.

[46] Levine SM. A survey of clinical practice of lung transplantation in North America. Chest 2004;125(4):1224–38.

[47] Gandhi MK, Khanna R. Human cytomegalovirus: clinical aspects, immune regulation, and emerging treatments. Lancet Infect Dis 2004;4:725–38.

[48] Rubin RH. Impact of cytomegalovirus infection on organ transplant recipients. Rev Infect Dis 1990;12(Suppl 7):S754–66.

[49] Limaye AP, Bakthavatsalam R, Kim HW, et al. Late-onset cytomegalovirus disease in liver transplant recipients despite antiviral prophylaxis. Transplantation 2004;78(9):1390–6.

[50] Zamora MR. Cytomegalovirus and lung transplantation. Am J Transplant 2004;4: 1219–26.

[51] Zamora MR, Davis RD, Leonard C. Management of cytomegalovirus infection in lung transplant recipients: evidence-based recommendations. Transplantation 2005;80(2): 157–63.

[52] van den Berg AP, Klompmaker IJ, Haagsma EB, et al. Evidence for an increased rate of bacterial infections in liver transplant patients with cytomegalovirus infection. Clin Transplant 1996;10:224–31.

[53] Falagas ME, Snydman DR, Griffith J, et al. Exposure to cytomegalovirus from the donated organ is a risk factor for bacteremia in orthotopic liver transplant recipients. Clin Infect Dis 1996;23:468–74.

[54] Falagas M, Snydman D, Griffith J, et al. Effect of cytomegalovirus infection status on first-year mortality rates among orthotopic liver transplant recipients. Ann Intern Med 1997; 126:275–9.

[55] Paya C, Humar A, Dominguez E, et al. Efficacy and safety of valganciclovir vs. oral ganciclovir for prevention of cytomegalovirus disease in solid organ transplant recipients. Am J Transplant 2004;4:611–20.

[56] Gane E, Saliba F, Valdecasas GJC, et al. Randomized trial of efficacy and safety of oral ganciclovir in the prevention of cytomegalovirus disease in liver-transplant recipients. Lancet 1997;350:1729–33.

[57] Weill D, Lock BJ, Wewers DL, et al. Combination prophylaxis with ganciclovir and cytomegalovirus (CMV) immune globulin after lung transplantation: effective CMV prevention following Daclizumab induction. Am J Transplant 2003;3(4):492–6.

[58] Aguado JM, Gomez-Sanchez MA, Lumbreras C, et al. Prospective randomized trial of efficacy of ganciclovir versus that of anti-cytomegalovirus (CMV) immunoglobulin to prevent CMV disease in CMV-seropositive heart transplant recipients treated with OKT3. Antimicrob Agents Chemother 1995;39(7):1643–5.

[59] Kalil AC, Levitsky J, Lyden E, et al. Meta-analysis: the efficacy of strategies to prevent organ disease by cytomegalovirus in solid organ transplant recipients. Ann Inter Med 2005; 143(12):870–80.

[60] Taber DJ, Ashcraft E, Baillie GM, et al. Valganciclovir prophylaxis in patients at high risk for the development of cytomegalovirus disease. Transpl Infect Dis 2004;6:101–9.

[61] Egan JJ, Lomax J, Barber L, et al. Preemptive treatment for the prevention of cytomegalovirus disease in lung and heart transplant recipients. Transplantation 1998;65(5):747–52.

[62] Sagedal S, Nordal KP, Hartmann A, et al. A prospective study of the natural course of cytomegalovirus infection and disease in renal allograft recipients. Transplantation 2000; 70(8):1166–74.

[63] Paya C, Wilson J, Espy M, et al. Preemptive use of oral ganciclovir to prevent cytomegalovirus infection in liver transplant patients: a randomized, placebo-controlled trial. J Infect Dis 2002;185:854–60.

[64] Limaye AP, Raghu G, Koelle DM, et al. High incidence of ganciclovir-resistant cytomegalovirus Infection among lung transplant recipients receiving preemptive therapy. J Infect Dis 2002;185:20–7.

[65] Boivin G, Goyette N, Gilbert C, et al. Clinical impact of ganciclovir-resistant cytomegalovirus infections in solid organ transplant patients. Transpl Infect Dis 2005;7(3–4):166–70.

[66] Singh N, Paterson DL. Aspergillus infections in transplant recipients. Clin Micro Rev 2005; 18:44–69.

[67] Panackal AA, Dahlman A, Keil KT, et al. Outbreak of invasive aspergillosis among renal transplant recipients. Transplantation 2003;75:1050–3.

[68] Herbrecht R, Denning DW, Patterson TF, et al. Voriconazole versus amphotericin B for primary therapy of invasive aspergillosis. N Engl J Med 2002;347:408–15.

[69] Minari A, Husni R, Avery RK, et al. The incidence of invasive aspergillosis among solid organ transplant recipients and implications for prophylaxis in lung transplants. Transpl Infect Dis 2002;4:195–200.

[70] Husain S, Alexander BD, Munoz P, et al. Opportunistic mycelial fungal infections in organ transplant recipients: emerging importance of non-*Aspergillus* mycelial fungi. Clin Infect Dis 2003;37:221–9.

[71] Kramer MR, Stoehr C, Lewiston NJ, et al. Trimethoprim-sulfamethoxazole prophylaxis for *Pneumocystis carinii* infections in heart-lung and lung transplantation—how effective and for how long? Transplantation 1992;53:586–9.

[72] Saigenji H, Kaneko M, Rhenmen B, et al. *Pneumocystis carinii* pneumonia after heart transplantation. Ann Thorac Surg 1991;52:107–11.

[73] Ng VL, Yajko DM, Hadley WK. Extrapulmonary pneumocystosis. Clin Micro Rev 1997; 10:401–18.

[74] Gordon SM, LaRosa SP, Kalmadi S, et al. Should prophylaxis for *Pneumocystis carinii* pneumonia in solid organ transplant recipients ever be discontinued? Clin Infect Dis 1999;28:240–6.

[75] Fishman JA. Prevention of infection caused by *Pneumocystis carinii* in transplant recipients. Clin Infect Dis 2001;33:1397–405.

[76] Stout JE, Yu VL. Legionellosis. N Engl J Med 1997;337:682–7.

[77] Kool JL, Fiore AE, Kioski CM, et al. More than 10 years of unrecognized nosocomial transmission of Legionnaires' disease among transplant patients. Infect Control Hosp Epidemiol 1998;19:898–904.

[78] Knirsch CA, Jakob K, Schoonmaker D, et al. An outbreak of *Legionella micdadei* pneumonia in transplant patients: evaluation, molecular epidemiology and control. Am J Med 2000;108:290–5.

[79] Tkatch LS, Kusne S, Irish WD, et al. Epidemiology of *Legionella* pneumonia and factors associated with *Legionella*-related mortality at a tertiary care center. Clin Infect Dis 1998;27:1479–86.

[80] Fraser TG, Zembower TR, Lynch P, et al. Cavitary *Legionella* pneumonia in a liver transplant recipient. Transpl Infect Dis 2004;6:77–80.

[81] Murdoch DR. Diagnosis of *Legionella* infection. Clin Infect Dis 2003;36:64–9.

[82] Ernst A, Gordon FD, Hayek J, et al. Lung abscess complicating *Legionella micdadei* pneumonia in an adult liver transplant recipient. Transplantation 1998;65:130–4.

[83] Ruskin J, Remington JS. Toxoplasmosis in the compromised host. Ann Intern Med 1976; 84:193–9.

[84] Renoult E, Georges E, Biava M-F, et al. Toxoplasmosis in kidney transplant recipients: report of six cases and review. Clin Infect Dis 1997;24:625–34.

[85] Mayes JT, O'Connor BJ, Avery R, et al. Transmission of *Toxoplasma gondii* infection by liver transplantation. Clin Infect Dis 1995;21:511–5.

[86] Ponticellli C, Campise MR. Neurological complications of kidney transplant recipients. J Nephrol 2005;18:521–8.

[87] Wulf MWH, vanCrevel R, Portier R, et al. Toxoplasmosis after renal transplantation: implications of a missed diagnosis. J Clin Microbiol 2005;43:3544–7.

[88] Munir A, Zaman M, Eltorky M. *Toxoplasma gondii* pneumonia in a pancreas transplant patient. South Med J 2000;93:614–7.

[89] Mitchell TG, Perfect JR. Cryptococcosis in the era of AIDS—100 years after the discovery of *Cryptococcus neoformans*. Clin Microbiol Rev 1995;8:515–48.

[90] Vilchez RA, Fung J, Kusne S. Cryptococcosis in organ transplant recipients: an overview. Am J Transplant 2002;2:575–80.

[91] Nosanchuk JD, Shoham S, Fries BC, et al. Evidence of zoonotic transmission of *Cryptococcus neoformans* from a pet cockatoo to an immunocompromised patient. Ann Intern Med 2000;132:205–8.

[92] Husain S, Wagener MM, Singh N. *Cryptococcus neoformans* infection in organ transplant recipients: variables influencing clinical characteristics and outcome. Emerg Infect Dis 2001;7:375–81.

[93] Wu G, Vilchez RA, Eidelman B, et al. Cryptococcal meningitis: an analysis among 5521 consecutive organ transplant recipients. Transpl Infect Dis 2002;4:183–8.

[94] Carlson KC, Mehlmauer M, Evans S, et al. Cryptococcal cellulitis in renal transplant recipients. J Am Acad Dermatol 1987;17:469–72.

[95] Singh N, Gayowski T, Wagener MM, et al. Clinical spectrum of invasive cryptococcosis in liver transplant recipients receiving tacrolimus. Clinical Transplantation 1997;11:66–70.

[96] Baumgarten KL, Valentine VG, Garcia-Diaz JB. Primary cutaneous cryptococcosis in a lung transplant recipient. South Med J 2004;97:692–5.

[97] Stamm AM, Dismukes WE, Simmons BP, et al. Listeriosis in renal transplant recipients: report of an outbreak and review of 102 cases. Rev Infect Dis 1982;4(3):665–82.

[98] Stamm AM, Smith SH, Kriklin JK, et al. Listerial myocarditis in cardiac transplantation. Rev Infect Dis 1990;12:820–3.

[99] Algan M, Jonon B, George JL, et al. *Listeria monocytogenes* endophthalmitis in a renal transplant patient receiving ciclosporin. Ophthalmologica 1990;201:23–7.

[100] Vargas V, Alemán C, deTorres I, et al. *Listeria monocytogenes*-associated acute hepatitis in a liver transplant recipient. Liver 1998;18:213–5.

[101] Sands M, Brown RB. Interactions of cyclosporine with antimicrobial agents. Rev Infect Dis 1989;11(5):691–7.

[102] Husain S, Singh N. The impact of novel immunosuppressive agents on infections in organ transplant recipients and the interactions of these agents with antimicrobials. Clin Infect Dis 2002;35(1):53–61.

[103] Anonymous. Immunosuppressive drug interactions with anti-infective agents. Am J Transplant 2004;4(Supp 10):164–8.

ELSEVIER
SAUNDERS

SURGICAL
CLINICS OF
NORTH AMERICA

Surg Clin N Am 86 (2006) 1147–1166

# The Preoperative Evaluation of the Transplanted Patient for Nontransplant Surgery

## Reginald Y. Gohh, MD*, Greg Warren, DO

*Division of Renal Diseases, Rhode Island Hospital, Brown University School of Medicine, 593 Eddy Street, APC-921, Providence, Rhode Island 02903, USA*

Refinements in immunosuppressive therapy and the medical management of organ transplant recipients have resulted in significant improvements in both short- and long-term outcomes. This has led to a dramatic increase in the number of individuals undergoing transplantation worldwide. In the United States alone, over 28,000 individuals received solid-organ transplants in 2005 [1]. With increasing success, there has been an increased willingness to transplant individuals previously felt to be unsuitable for such procedures. Factors such as age and various medical comorbidities are no longer considered contraindications to transplantation, and hence, an increasing number of recipients may require medical care not specifically related to the transplant. At some point, these patients may require elective or emergent surgery, making it important for all surgeons to be familiar with the factors that may influence surgical outcomes in transplanted patients, along with issues that are likely to affect optimal timing of surgery and postoperative care. Most transplant centers use a team approach to managing these complex patients, relying on medical professionals experienced in the care and management of these individuals. Close interaction with the transplant team is likely the single most important step in preparing the transplanted patient for surgery and managing their postoperative care. This article will summarize factors important in the preoperative evaluation of transplanted individuals, with particular emphasis on medical comorbidities, and discuss some of the organ specific issues related to various solid organ recipients.

* Corresponding author.
*E-mail address:* rgohh@lifespan.org (R.Y. Gohh).

0039-6109/06/$ - see front matter © 2006 Elsevier Inc. All rights reserved.
doi:10.1016/j.suc.2006.07.001
*surgical.theclinics.com*

## General considerations

The overall management of surgical disease in transplant recipients generally adheres to the same fundamental principles of sound operative care appropriate to all surgical illnesses. However, it is important to remember that these patients are chronically immunosuppressed. Although most stable transplant recipients achieve excellent functional capacities and are able to live normal productive lives, they are at increased risk for infectious complications, and may present clinically in a different fashion from their immunocompetent counterparts. This may sometimes result in serious underestimation of disease severity. Accordingly, a high level of vigilance is paramount, and occasionally it may become necessary to proceed with exploratory surgery to establish a firm diagnosis. Furthermore, one must consider the potential impact of any operative procedure on transplant organ function. Because many of these transplanted organs have diminished reserve when compared with average patients, even modest intraoperative insults such as hypotension may have deleterious consequences on transplant organ function. For these reasons, when provided with two or more options, a cautious surgical approach, staged procedures, and minimally invasive options are often preferred in these patients.

An important component of the pretransplant surgical clearance is to formulate a plan for the management of immunosuppression in the perioperative period. In general, the maintenance of oral immunosuppressive medication is preferred whenever possible. From a practical perspective, this may be difficult to achieve in clinical situations where gastrointestinal absorption is compromised. These include scenarios involving surgical ileus, small bowel obstruction, or increased gastrointestinal motility (eg, diarrhea). In these situations, temporary conversion to intravenous formulations is acceptable with appropriate dose adjustments for increased drug bioavailability. Cyclosporine, tacrolimus, mycophenolate mofetil, azathioprine, and corticosteroids are all available as intravenous preparations. Sirolimus is not clinically available in parental form and, accordingly, this drug is usually transiently discontinued when oral administration is not feasible.

In life-threatening situations, it is occasionally necessary to temporarily discontinue immunosuppression in the hope that a more robust immune system may permit resolution of an acute medical problem. This strategy would be indicated in clinical situations such as severe infections that are not responding to usual aggressive measures. Although specific guidelines are lacking for the management of such transplant recipients, multiple anecdotal case reports suggest that septic transplant patients can be maintained off all immunosuppressive therapy up to several months without risking rejection, perhaps due to the differential expression of various cytokines (IL-10, gamma-interferon) that may have rejection-sparing effects [2]. However, the clinical course must be followed closely when such a decision is made, and immunosuppression reintroduced with clinical recovery to avoid acute allograft rejection. Clearly, such a decision is highly subjective, and this issue emphasizes the importance of close coordination with an experienced transplant team.

## Cardiac evaluation

Cardiovascular disease (CVD) complications are a major cause of morbidity and mortality among organ transplant recipients. The risk of CVD is particularly pronounced in renal transplant recipients, where the incidence of CVD is nearly twice that of the general population and is the leading cause of death in these individuals [3]. Among younger patients the effect is even more striking, with a 10-fold increase in CVD-related mortality for kidney transplant recipients less than 45 years of age [3]. Because most pancreas transplant recipients often suffer from concomitant renal insufficiency, they fall into a similar risk category. Congestive heart failure is also a common condition among recipients following kidney transplantation and, in particular, its de novo occurrence has been associated with poor patient survival [4]. Hence, perhaps the most pressing concern for any patient undergoing surgery is the risk of a perioperative cardiovascular event.

The elevated risk of CVD in kidney transplant recipients is due to a variety of factors, including the negative impact of chronic kidney failure on the cardiovascular system, and the association of end-stage renal disease (ESRD) with multiple cardiovascular risk factors [5]. Not surprisingly, a prior history of ischemic heart disease, common among all ESRD patients, is a major risk factor for a CVD following transplantation [6]. Established risk factors for the development of CVD such as hypertension, hyperlipidemia, physical inactivity, metabolic syndrome, obesity, and diabetes are extremely prevalent in this population, and are not necessarily cured by transplantation [6]. Therefore, by the time many prospective recipients receive a kidney transplant, they have already suffered extensive damage to their cardiovascular systems, and should be considered at high risk for CVD and treated accordingly.

Additionally, variables specific to the posttransplant setting, such as some immunosuppressive drugs and acute rejection episodes, can worsen or create new cardiovascular risk factors. Calcineurin inhibitors, such as cyclosporine and tacrolimus, and corticosteroids have been associated with an increased risk of developing hypertension, lipid abnormalities, and diabetes [7]. Likewise, the hyperlipidemic effects of sirolimus have also been well documented, and a significant proportion of patients maintained on this agent have required long-term lipid lowering therapy [8]. Note that these complications of immunosuppression are common to all organ transplant recipients, and cardiovascular complications in nonrenal transplant recipients are also likely to become more common with longer follow-up and improved graft survival.

Because of the high prevalence of CVD, along with the desire to avoid transplanting patients at high risk of death, the majority of patients pursuing transplantation undergo an extensive cardiovascular evaluation. The American Society of Transplantation recommends the following approach to patients undergoing evaluation for kidney transplantation: patients over the age of 50 and all diabetic patients should have an exercise tolerance test, while patients with abnormal EKGs or those who have smoked for > 5 years also should undergo stress testing [9,10]. The guidelines also advocate cardiac catheterization, with the goal of correcting significant stenosis, for those with reversible ischemia and diabetics with any suggestion of an abnormal test. Because the morbidity and mortality of both lung and liver transplantation are increased in patients with underlying coronary artery disease, similarly stringent cardiac evaluations are performed in the potential recipients of these organs [11,12]. Records of these cardiac evaluations should be easily obtainable from the patient's transplant center or cardiologist.

An obvious question that arises is how long a negative workup should be relied upon, without performing additional testing before surgery. This decision needs be addressed on an individual basis, and should not only take into consideration the patient's symptoms and present functional capacity, but also the risk associated with the specific surgery in mind. As with any preoperative evaluation, a thorough history of cardiac symptoms should be elicited, with one caveat being that many diabetic patients have asymptomatic coronary disease. Again, it is important to stress that transplantation does not reverse preexisting cardiovascular disease, and that previously present risk factors may be compounded by new ones, making cardiovascular disease a very high probability in many transplanted individuals. To emphasize this further, a recent epidemiologic study of cardiovascular disease after renal transplantation demonstrated a progressive increase in the incidences of ischemic heart disease, cerebrovascular disease, and peripheral vascular disease. Specifically, 23% developed new-onset ischemic heart disease, 15% had a major cerebrovascular event, and 15% developed peripheral vascular disease [7].

Given the high probability of cardiovascular disease in these individuals, their perioperative management attains equal importance. Preoperative β-blockers have been shown to be effective in preventing cardiovascular events in high-risk individuals and, unless otherwise contraindicated, should be prescribed liberally in this population [13]. Likewise, postoperative hypertension should be aggressively managed, and can often be handled by maintaining patients on their previous antihypertensive agents. Given the high incidence of left ventricular dysfunction in this population, avoidance of overaggressive fluid resuscitation can help prevent complications such as pulmonary edema and volume overload.

## Level of immunosuppression and risk of postsurgical infection

Infection is an inevitable consequence of life-long immunosuppression. Unfortunately, no single test is widely available that can reliably predict a patient's overall level of immunosuppression and subsequent risk of rejection or infection. However, long-term clinical experience has allowed for the categorization of patients into risk groups that help to predict their susceptibility to infection. With the standardization of immunosuppressive protocols, a pattern or "timetable" has emerged that not only helps predict when infections occur, but the types of pathogens most likely to be involved as well [14]. This pattern of susceptibility tends to follow the "net state of immunosuppression," which is influenced greatly not only by the dose, but also by the duration, nature, and temporal sequence of immunosuppressive therapy. For instance, because the risk of acute rejection is highest in the first weeks to months following transplantation, immunosuppression is maintained at high levels in this period and tapered to maintenance dosages thereafter. Similarly, acute rejection is usually managed with high-dose steroids or antilymphocyte antibody therapy (for steroid-resistant rejection), followed by an intensification of maintenance immunosuppressive therapy to levels often equal to or even greater than the initial 6-month perioperative period. Both of these clinical scenarios represent periods of heightened risk for infection, and hence, a suboptimal time to proceed with an elective or nonemergent surgery. Note that certain viral infections, such as cytomegalovirus (CMV), are themselves immunosuppressive, and may further increase the risk of secondary infections. A history of recent infection should at least prompt request for advice from the transplant team regarding optimal timing for surgery.

As with any patient undergoing an invasive procedure, antibiotic prophylaxis is an important component of the perioperative management of the transplant recipient. Although these patients may be considered at higher risk of developing infectious complications after surgical, endoscopic, or dental procedures, there is no evidence to suggest that prolonged or heightened antibiotic prophylaxis has any added benefit in preventing infectious complications in these individuals. For this reason, we recommend adherence to the antimicrobial guidelines proposed by the Medicare National Surgical Infection Prevention Project, with therapy tailored according to the expected risk of contamination [15]. However, given the frequent unusual clinical presentations of these patients, we do advocate the liberal use of cultures if there is any possibility of an infectious etiology. Oral amoxicillin or clindamycin are appropriate for dental procedures, whereas broader spectrum coverage to include Gram-positive and Gram-negative bacteria is warranted for intraabdominal procedures. It is recommended that infusion of the first antimicrobial dose be given within 1 to 2 hours before the surgical incision, because these patients have lower rates of surgical site infection compared with patients who receive them either too early or postoperatively.

**Tissue integrity and wound healing**

Virtually all transplant recipients will experience the delayed development of tensile strength due to the effects of immunosuppression and underlying systemic illness on wound healing. Glucocorticoids, even at low doses, have been associated with impaired tissue integrity, leading to enhanced friability of skin, superficial blood vessels and the intestinal wall [16,17]. Cautious handling of tissues is thus particularly important in these patients to avoid wound-healing complications. Many transplant surgeons advocate the use of nonabsorbable sutures whenever possible. When an absorbable suture is warranted, monofilament, synthetic, absorbable sutures have been recommended because of their ability to maintain adequate tensile strength over a long period. Due to concerns of delayed wound healing, it also has been recommended that skin staples be kept in place two to three times longer in the transplant recipient.

More recently, the use of the immunosuppressive agent sirolimus has been associated with detrimental effects on wound healing, even during the immediate posttransplantation period. In a recent study comparing sirolimus to tacrolimus as a primary immunosuppressive therapy, the incidence of allograft wound complications (including perigraft fluid collections, superficial wound infections, and incisional hernias) was significantly higher in the former group [18]. Whether or not these adverse cutaneous effects persist with prolonged use of this agent during subsequent surgeries is not well studied, but should be considered when embarking on surgery in a patient maintained on this agent.

### Adrenal insufficiency

Because most transplant recipients are maintained on chronic corticosteroids as part of their immunosuppressive regimen, the possibility of adrenal insufficiency is often raised when these patients develop emergent problems requiring surgical intervention. Fortunately, current doses of steroids used for routine maintenance immunosuppression have been markedly reduced compared with previous standards (usually 5–10 mg of prednisone), making adrenal suppression much less of an issue. Although the penalty associated with the temporary administration of "stress dose" corticosteroids would be seemingly small, such therapy is not entirely benign, and occasionally can be associated with gastritis, bleeding, and the induction or worsening of diabetes. Furthermore, there is sufficient evidence to suggest the administration of these high doses is usually unnecessary. In a prospective study of 40 renal transplant patients admitted with various sources of stress (including sepsis, metabolic abnormalities, and surgery), no clinical evidence of adrenal insufficiency was noted despite being maintained only on their baseline dose of prednisone (5–10 mg/d) [19]. Additionally, the study demonstrated that the cosyntropin stimulation test significantly overestimated the presence of clinically significant adrenal deficiency, and hence, was not a reliable marker for the need of additional glucocorticoids. For this reason, several authors have recommended that patients on chronic low-dose glucocorticoids undergoing surgery receive only their usual dose of gluco-corticoid perioperatively [19–21]. In contrast, patients who have received more than 20 mg/d of prednisone or its equivalent for more than 3 weeks should be assumed to have functional suppression of the hypothalamic–pituitary–adrenal axis, but nevertheless, rarely require additional steroids to accommodate acute stress [22].

However, if the patient exhibits signs or symptoms of adrenal insuffi-ciency postoperatively, the use of perioperative "stress coverage" would be warranted. Although traditionally the dosage used for stress coverage has been 100 mg of hydrocortisone every 8 hours, this dose in actuality is far higher than the physiologic cortisol response, which peaks at 150 mg/d after major surgery and returns quickly to baseline. A consensus paper recommends giving much lower peak doses (maximum 50 mg of hy-drocortisone every 8 hours with dose adjustment based on the degree of sur-gical stress), and then quickly returning the dosage to baseline [23]. This strategy is designed to parallel the physiologic response of the normal adre-nal gland to surgical stress. There is no evidence to suggest that steroid sup-plementation needs to be tapered over a prolonged period. A taper over 1 to 3 days is adequate in uncomplicated situations, and this helps to minimize any adverse effects of high-dose steroids.

## Thrombophilia

The early posttransplant period is associated with an increased risk of vascular complications such as arterial and venous thrombosis of the allo-graft, often with catastrophic consequences and eventual loss of the trans-planted organ. Allograft thrombosis has been attributed to such factors as technical complications, endothelial injury, and the unique tenuous blood supply of the transplanted organs (especially liver and pancreas grafts). However, mounting evidence in renal transplant recipients points to throm-bophilic conditions as the underlying etiology in the majority of early throm-botic events after transplant surgery. Acquired coagulation defects are particularly common in patients with ESRD. Antiphospholipid antibodies and elevated serum homocysteine levels are highly prevalent in this popula-tion [24,25]. For this reason, screening for thrombophilia should be consid-ered in ESRD patients with a clinical history of thromboembolic events (deep vein thrombosis, early or frequent arteriovenous (AV) fistula thrombosis, clotting of the dialysis filter, for example). Testing usually includes screening for antiphospholipid antibodies, mutations of factor V Leiden or the pro-thrombin gene, and clotting factor deficiencies. The presence of antiphospho-lipid antibodies and a history of thrombosis constitute the antiphospholipid antibody syndrome and define a population at particularly high risk. Perio-perative anticoagulation in such identified patients has been shown to reduce the risk of renal allograft thrombosis. Although the optimal management of thrombophilic states in renal transplantation remains unclear, it has been our practice to continue anticoagulation for a minimum of 6 months. These factors need to be taken into consideration when transplant patients present for elective or emergency surgery to ensure that they receive adequate prophylaxis.

In contrast, liver transplant recipients may experience thrombocytopenia (secondary to hypersplenism) that may persist into the postoperative period. The thrombocytopenia is usually of no clinical significance, although the dosage of either azathioprine or mycophenolate mofetil may need to be reduced due to their marrow suppressive effects. Platelet transfusions occasionally may be necessary to avoid bleeding complications during surgical procedures. Nevertheless, the consequences of hypersplenism generally resolve after successful liver transplantation and rarely present long-term problems.

## Organ-specific considerations

### Kidney transplant recipients

Like dialysis, transplantation generally falls short of replacing normal kidney function. Although many renal transplant recipients have serum creatinine levels within the normal range, the average glomerular filtration rate of kidney transplant recipients rarely exceeds 50 mL/min/1.73 m$^2$ (based on an equation derived from the Modification of Diet in Renal Disease study) [26]. Therefore, kidney transplant recipients are often exposed to the same variables of abnormal renal function found in all patients with chronic kidney disease. From a surgical standpoint, there must be an increased awareness not only for the potential for fluid and electrolyte abnormalities, but also the diminished ability to normally metabolize or excrete different anesthetics or analgesics, leading to toxic accumulation of these agents. For instance, the free fraction of thiopental may be doubled in renal failure, resulting in exaggerated clinical effects and the need for dose adjustment [27]. For this reason, it seems wise to choose drugs that do not rely on renal excretion such as propofol and atracurium. A similar strategy should be used when choosing postoperative analgesics and sedatives. In particular, meperidine and propoxyphene should be avoided in patients with significant graft dysfunction [28]. Although both agents undergo hepatic metabolism, their metabolites have prolonged half-lives in patients with renal insufficiency and have been associated with significant neurologic and cardiac toxicities, respectively. If an opiate is required for pain relief in these patients, fentanyl is likely best tolerated because of its short distribution phase, the lack of active metabolites, and unchanged free fraction [29].

Transient postoperative deterioration of renal function is relatively common and is chiefly due to alterations in renal perfusion. Because transplanted kidneys are functionally denervated, they may lose their innate ability to autoregulate renal blood flow, and hence, may be more sensitive to sudden changes in blood pressure. For this reason, medications that may adversely affect renal plasma flow or have the potential for nephrotoxicity should be avoided if possible. Nonsteroidal anti-inflammatory drugs should not be used for this reason. Conversely, neither diuretics nor intravenous fluids should be given without an initial thorough evaluation of the patient's volume status. Accordingly, proper management may require right heart monitoring to provide objective parameters for intravascular volume management.

Note that chronic renal insufficiency has also emerged as a significant problem in the recipients of other solid organs, perhaps reflecting the improved long-term survival of these individuals. The exact incidence of chronic kidney disease in this population varies depending on the definition applied, but it is estimated that at least 18% of liver recipients, 32% of heart recipients, and 20% of lung recipients will experience some degree of renal insufficiency at 5 years [30]. It is estimated that up to 29% of these individuals will eventually progress to end-stage renal disease and require renal replacement therapy [30]. The nephrotoxicity associated with the long-term use of the calcineurin inhibitors, cyclosporine and tacrolimus, has been implicated as a major contributor to this problem. The same perioperative considerations outlined above should be applied to nonrenal transplant patients with renal impairment.

## Liver transplant recipients

Successful orthotopic liver transplantation negates the detrimental effects of end-stage liver disease on multiple organ systems, and nearly complete rehabilitation can be anticipated in the majority of surviving patients. Although transaminases are generally elevated in the immediate postoperative period, these and other tests of synthetic liver function gradually return to normal over the first 2 weeks. Interestingly, recovery of the ability for drug metabolism occurs almost immediately after reperfusion of the graft, and substantial capacity to metabolize hepatically cleared agents such as morphine has been reported [31]. The presence of persistent hyperbilirubinemia or coagulopathy indicates severe organ dysfunction, and should prompt postponement of all but emergent surgery.

The usual hemodynamic profile of patients with end-stage liver disease is one of hyperdynamic circulation with systemic vasodilatation. This may result from a number of factors, including vasodilators released into the systemic circulation from the splanchnic vascular bed and the development of peripheral resistance to vasoconstrictors such as norepinephrine and angiotensin II [32]. Liver transplantation results in the successful reversal of this hyperdynamic state, and cardiac performance improves in the months after transplantation [31].

However, several unique factors that impair oxygenation and ventilation in patients with end-stage liver disease make them more susceptible to pulmonary dysfunction in the posttransplant period. Intrapulmonary shunting resulting in hypoxemia may occur as a result of the hepatopulmonary syndrome [33]. Ventilation/perfusion mismatch can occur as a result of pleural effusions, ascites, and diaphragmatic dysfunction. Diffusion abnormalities have also been described, and may be due to interstitial pneumonitis or pulmonary hypertension [31,33]. Fortunately, oxygenation usually improves after transplantation in the majority of patients, although this may take months in advanced cases [34]. However, significant hypoxemia from intrapulmonary shunting may require more time to achieve reversal of the underlying pathology, and in some cases hypoxia may not resolve at all [35].

Some anesthetic concerns deserve particular attention. Because of its denervated state, the normal physiologic mechanisms that maintain hepatic blood flow may be impaired following transplantation, making the allograft more prone to ischemic injury [36]. Hence, the administration of volatile anesthetics may theoretically decrease hepatic blood flow resulting in allograft dysfunction. By decreasing portal resistance, isoflurane may actually improve portal blood flow and should be considered the volatile anesthetic of choice [37]. Alternatively, the use of regional anesthesia or analgesia may also be considered if the setting permits. Note that there is no evidence to suggest an increased risk of developing hepatitis after the administration of inhaled anesthetics in liver transplant recipients [38,39].

It is important to maintain the intravascular volume and systemic blood pressure during surgery in these individuals. Drugs such as cimetidine and propranolol that may decrease hepatic blood flow should be used judiciously, if at all. By increasing splanchnic vascular resistance, hypoxia, hypercapnia, excessive positive end expiratory pressure, and high airway pressures can also contribute to impaired hepatic perfusion [37].

## Lung transplant recipients

Lung transplantation has emerged over the past 20 years as a successful therapeutic intervention for a variety of end-stage pulmonary parenchymal and vascular diseases. The most common indications for lung transplantation include chronic obstructive pulmonary disease (COPD), emphysema due to alpha-1 antitrypsin deficiency, idiopathic pulmonary fibrosis, and cystic fibrosis [38]. Treatment options include single lung transplantation, bilateral lung transplantation, and combined heart–lung transplantation. Despite the limitations of lung transplantation, the majority of patients benefit from this therapy. Patients who were previously totally disabled, unable to carry out activities of daily living without enormous difficulty, are usually able to resume active lifestyles. With improved life expectancies, it is likely that an increasing number of these patients will present for nontransplant procedures and surgeries.

Patients with lung transplants often require several months before they reach their peak expected lung capacity. During these first few months, factors such as pain, altered chest wall mechanics, acute lung injury, and respiratory muscle dysfunction can all diminish allograft function [37]. Although bilateral transplantation eventually results in normal pulmonary function, the efficacy of single lung transplantation will depend on the severity of the underlying disease and compromise of the remaining native lung. Nevertheless, arterial oxygenation usually returns to normal without the need for supplemental oxygenation by the time of hospital discharge. In a similar fashion, hypercapnea (secondary to a blunted ventilatory response to carbon dioxide) in patients with emphysema normalizes within a few weeks following transplantation [40]. Despite these functional improvements, peak oxygen consumption, and hence peak exercise performance, does not return to normal values after transplant, especially in recipients of single lung transplants [41].

The lung is the only allograft exposed to the external environment and, as such, is particularly prone to complications of both infection and rejection [42]. Clinically, it is very difficult to differentiate between these two entities. For instance, bronchiolitis obliterans, the pathogenic expression of chronic rejection in lung transplants, can mimic the symptoms of an upper respiratory infection. These concerns heighten the importance of a thorough preoperative evaluation, which should include a careful history of functional capacity (exercise capacity, need for supplemental oxygen) and the presence of symptoms such as dyspnea, fatigue, fevers, or sputum production. It is also recommended that these patients routinely undergo objective testing such as pulmonary function testing, chest radiographs, and arterial blood gases, with results compared with previous values to help detect new or worsening lung dysfunction [43]. Any suggestion of or trend toward deterioration should delay all nonemergent surgery until both rejection and infection can be excluded.

A number of interesting physiologic changes have been observed following lung transplantation that may potentially impact the outcomes of nontransplant surgeries. Many of these reflect the effects of pulmonary denervation distal to the bronchial anastomosis. In single-lung transplant recipients, the carinal receptors remain intact and their stimulation elicits a cough reflex [44]. In contrast, patients with a tracheal anastomosis lose the cough reflex and are more prone to retention of secretions and silent aspiration [45]. Although denervation appears to have minimal effects on the pattern of breathing, mucociliary transport is also impaired and airway hyperresponsiveness leading to bronchospasm is common [46,47]. Given these considerations, incentive spirometry, chest physiotherapy and secretion mobilization are important in the perioperative setting to promote pulmonary hygiene.

Lung transplantation also results in disruption of the pulmonary lymphatics and bronchial circulation, leading to an increased risk of pulmonary edema. Although the lymphatics do show evidence of reforming, the extent and timing are unclear [48]. Therefore, fluid management should be conservative in the perioperative setting and diuretics prescribed if necessary.

Another issue pertinent to recipients of single lung transplants is that the majority of blood flow and ventilation (60–80%) is directed toward the allograft; hence, hypoxemia may ensue if the patient is placed in the lateral position, especially if the allograft is in the dependent position [49].

A few anesthetic concerns with lung transplant recipients deserve particular emphasis. If general anesthesia is required, airway management can be challenging, and the anesthesiologist needs to be aware of the possibility for altered upper airway anatomy. In single-lung transplant recipients, an emphysematous native lung will be highly compliant and at risk for dynamic hyperinflation, whereas the allograft will have low to normal compliance. Therefore, positive pressure ventilation may induce compression of the transplanted lung [37]. In contrast, high airway pressures are required when the patient's native lung demonstrates restrictive physiology, as in pulmonary fibrosis. Distribution of this high-pressure flow to the lung allograft may then result in barotrauma and volutrauma. In these settings, placement of a double lumen tube for differential lung ventilation should be considered [50]. Regardless, in all lung transplantation cases caution should be exercised when considering the use of anxiolytic premedications that may blunt the respiratory drive, particularly in patients with marginal gas exchange or $CO_2$ retention. Further, given the above concerns, it may be argued that a regional anesthesia technique would be preferable to general anesthesia whenever possible to decrease the risk of airway trauma and aspiration [37].

## Heart transplant recipients

Cardiac transplantation has evolved as the treatment of choice for many patients with end-stage heart disease that remain severely disabled despite optimal medical therapy. Recent data from the registry of the International Society for Heart and Lung Transplantation suggest a gradual improvement in patient survival over the last 20 years, with the patient half-life now approaching 10 years [51]. Most patients who undergo orthotopic heart transplantation are able to achieve normal active lifestyles, regaining New York Heart Association Class I functional capacity [52].

As with lung transplants, the physiologic function of heart transplant recipients is complicated by the absence of autonomic enervation. The transplanted heart has no sympathetic, parasympathetic, or sensory enervation and functions independently of the reflexes mediated by these nervous systems. Hence, carotid sinus massage and the Valsalva maneuver have no effect on the heart rate [31]. Cardiac baroreflexes and the sympathetic response to laryngoscopy and tracheal intubation are lost for the same reason. Although denervation has little effect on resting allograft function, β-receptor density increases and myocyte sensitivity to circulating catecholamines is enhanced [31]. The basal resting heart rate is higher (typically 90–100 beats per minute) due to the absence of vagal tone [53]. Although myocardial catecholamine stores are completely depleted within days, intrinsic myocardial contractility remains unaffected. Therefore, the cardiac index is generally normal [54]. Left and right ventricular ejection fraction as well as stroke volume are also normal, and remain so over at least the first 5 years [55].

Two P waves are often seen on the electrocardiograph of the orthotopic heart transplant recipient, as a cuff of native atria containing the sinoatrial node is often left in place to permit surgical anastomosis to the grafted heart [37]. However, because the native P wave cannot cross the suture line, it has no influence on the chronotropic characteristics of the transplanted heart. Conduction abnormalities are common, occurring in 70% to 75% of patients [56,57]. These include hemiblocks (approximately 20%), right bundle branch block (40–50%), and left bundle branch block (5%). Permanent pacemakers are required in 5% to 10% of patients, and their proper function should be confirmed before proceeding with any surgical procedure [37]. The mode of the pacemaker may also need to be altered to prevent unwanted discharge during the use of electrocautery.

Despite refinements in immunosuppressive therapy, allograft rejection remains a leading cause of mortality in heart transplant recipients. Acute allograft rejection usually occurs within the first 6 months, and can only be reliably diagnosed by ventricular myocardial biopsy [58]. Although mild rejection does not compromise cardiac contractility, ongoing or severe rejection can result in significant systolic and diastolic dysfunction. Therefore, significant echocardiographic changes should prompt further evaluation before surgery. Chronic allograft rejection usually presents as accelerated coronary artery, and is the leading cause of death in long-standing cardiac recipients [59]. Interestingly, because of the absence of sensory enervation, heart transplant recipients may have significant myocardial ischemia without any clinical symptoms of angina.

An operative plan should take into account the altered pharmacodynamic effects of many drugs on the denervated cardiac allograft. For example, both epinephrine and norepinephrine have an augmented inotropic effect in heart transplant recipients, whereas dopamine is less effective in this regard [31,60]. Isoproterenol and dobutamine have similar efficacy in either denervated or normal hearts, and are effective inotropic agents in heart transplant recipients [31]. Other drug classes that act through the autonomic nervous system, such as anticholinergics, anticholinesterases, and some muscle relaxants, generally have minimal effects on the transplanted heart [37]. Table 1 and Box 1 summarize the pharmacologic effects of a number of these agents on the cardiac allograft.

Heart transplant recipients can be managed with any anesthetic technique [44,61]. However, because heart transplant recipients are preload dependent and are more prone to myocardial dysfunction, anesthetic agents with vasodilating properties and techniques that are more likely to result in hypotension should be avoided. For this reason, hemodynamic monitoring or transesophageal echocardiography may be useful to assess preload and

Table 1
Antimicrobial prophylaxis for selected surgical procedures

| Operation | Recommended antibiotic prophylaxis | Comments |
|---|---|---|
| Cardiothoracic surgery | Cefazolin, cefuroxime, or cefamandole; if patient has a B-lactam allergy: vancomycin or clindamycin | Most of the guidelines agree that prophylaxis for cardiac surgery should be administered for >24 hours after surgery. The ASHP suggests continuation of prophylaxis for cardiothoracic surgery up to 72 h; however, its authors suggest that prophylaxis for <24 h may be appropriate. Cefamanadole is not available in the U.S. |
| Vascular surgery | Cefazolin or cefuroxime; if patient has a B-lactam allergy: Vancomycin with or without gentamycin, or clindamycin | |
| Colon surgery | Oral: neomycin plus erythromycin base, or neomycin plus metronidazole; parenteral: cefoxitin or cefotetan, or cefazolin plus metronidazole | Currently, none of the guidelines address antimicrobial prophylaxis for those patients with B-lactam allergy. Cefmetazole is not available in the U.S. Although a recent study indicates that the combination of oral prophylaxis with parenteral antibiotics may result in lower wound infection rates, this is not specified in any of the published guidelines. |
| Hip or knee arthroplasty | Cefazolin or cefuroxime; if the patient has a B-lactam allergy: vancomycin or clindamycin | Although not addressed in any of the published guidelines, the workgroup recommends that prophylactic antimicrobial be completely infused before inflation of the tourniquet. Cefuroxime is recommended as a choice for patients undergoing total hip arthroplasty. |
| Vaginal or abdominal hysterectomy | Cefazolin, cefotetan, cefoxitin, or cefuroxime | Metronidazole monotherapy is recommended in the ACOG Practice Bulletin as an alternative to cephalosporin prophylaxis for patients undergoing hysterectomy. Trovafloxin, although still available in the U.S., is recommended only for serious infections. |

*Abbreviations:* ACOG, American College of Obstetricians and Gynecologists; ASHP, American Society of Health-System Pharmacists.

*Adapted from* Bratzler, DW, Houck, PM. Antimicrobial prophylaxis for surgery: an advisory statement from the national surgical prevention project. CID 2004;38:1706–15; with permission.

---

**Box 1. Effect of various medications on the transplanted heart**

*Drugs with minimal pharmacologic efficacy*
  Anticholinergics
    Atropine
    Glycopyrrolate
    Scopolamine
  Anticholinesterases
    Neostigmine[a]
    Edrophonium
    Pyridostigmine
  Paralytics (usually affect heart rate)
    Pancuronium
    Gallamine
    Physostigmine

*Drugs that retain pharmacologic efficacy*
  Isoproteranol
  Dobutamine
  Ephedrine
  Dopamine
  Glucagon
  Digoxin (inotropic effects only)
  Epinephrine (somewhat reduced)
  Norepinephrine (somewhat reduced)
  B-blockers
  Phosphodiesterase inhibitors

------
[a] May cause bradycardia

---

identifying ischemia, particularly in surgical procedures that involve large volume shifts. Some authors have advocated general anesthesia over regional anesthesia due to the potential for an impaired response to hypotension after spinal or epidural anesthesia [31]. Despite their well-known myocardial depressant properties, volatile agents are generally well tolerated as long as the patient is not in decompensated heart failure [37].

**Pancreas transplant recipients**

Pancreas transplantation is unique in that it has essentially a single indication—the treatment of diabetes mellitus (DM). Although the majority of pancreas transplant recipients suffer from type I DM, there has been an increased willingness in recent years to also offer transplantation to individuals with type II DM. Rarely, it has also been used for the prevention of diabetes that would result from total pancreatectomy. Pancreas transplantation also differs from other types of organ transplantation in that greater uncertainty exists as to whether the procedure is justified at all. It is not a life-sustaining procedure, and insulin treatment is a reasonable alternate therapy that is both relatively inexpensive and effective. Essentially, all pancreas transplantations currently require immunosuppressive therapy, and thus pancreas transplantation alone is a trade-off of insulin for immunosuppressive therapy. For this reason, pancreas transplantation has been reserved for "brittle" diabetics with frequent life-threatening complications or individuals who already require immunosuppressive therapy for a concomitant renal transplant (to treat diabetic nephropathy). The majority of pancreas transplants are therefore performed on those most severely affected by diabetes in which severe end-organ dysfunction is already established. Therefore, it should be assumed that the majority of these patients will have coronary artery disease and should undergo perioperative β-blockade unless otherwise contraindicated [62]. Many of these patients will have had a cardiac stress test or coronary angiogram performed previously, and these results should be reviewed before the patient undergoes any surgical procedure.

Pancreas transplantation effectively restores normal glucose metabolism, and may improve the lesions associated with diabetic neuropathy [63]. However, this process may take years to achieve and in a manner analogous to that of the transplanted heart, cardiovascular autonomic neuropathy in pancreas transplant recipients may result in a functionally denervated heart. This may manifest clinically as fluctuations in blood pressure with associated orthostasis, loss of beat-to-beat variability in heart rate, silent ischemia, and a blunted response to atropine [37]. Gastrointestinal autonomic neuropathy can result in disorders of esophageal motility and gastric emptying (gastroparesis), and may necessitate a rapid sequence induction or the application of cricoid pressure during anesthesia induction. Genitourinary autonomic neuropathy generally manifests as bladder dysfunction, which may result in an increased risk of urinary tract infections and difficultly voiding postoperatively.

Formal recommendations regarding the perioperative management of glucose levels in pancreas transplant recipients are not available, although clinical experience indicates that these individuals usually do not require supplemental insulin to compensate for the stress of surgery. Similarly, the effects of anesthesia on the catecholamine and glucagon response to hypoglycemia have not been well studied, but in general, counterregulatory mechanisms improve following successful pancreas transplantation [64]. However, in patients with failed pancreas grafts, the management of glucose levels, acid-base status, and electrolytes should be handled similarly to that of any diabetic patient. It should be noted that severe, refractory metabolic acidosis might occur during the bladder drainage of the exocrine pancreas transplants due to large bicarbonate losses [65].

## Summary

As greater numbers of people enjoy the success of modern transplantation, the need to optimally manage nontransplant surgical disease has become increasingly apparent. The fundamental principles of surgery continue to apply, but it is important to recognize that differences do exist between these chronically immunosuppressed individuals and the general population. Transplant recipients have unquestionably more medical problems, particularly in regard to cardiovascular disease, and function day after day with a precarious functional reserve. Therefore, it is essential that surgeons involved in the care of these patients develop a clear understanding of the physiology of the transplanted organ, the pharmacology of the immunosuppressive drugs, and the underlying surgical conditions to be remedied. Because most practicing surgeons will encounter only a few transplant recipients within their practice, close collaboration with the transplant team is recommended. Recent experience demonstrates that with a multidisciplinary approach, appropriate preoperative evaluation and attention to detail surgeons can anticipate excellent outcomes for this challenging group of patients.

## References

[1] Organ Procurement and Transplantation Network. Available at: www.optn.org. Accessed March 1, 2006.
[2] Burke GW, Ciancio G, Cirocco R, et al. Association of interleukin-10 with rejection-sparing effect in septic kidney transplant recipients. Transplantation 1996;61:1114–6.
[3] Foley RN, Parfrey PS, Sarnak MJ. Clinical epidemiology of cardiovascular disease in chronic renal disease. Am J Kidney Dis 1998;32:S112–9.
[4] Lentine KL, Schnitzler MA, Abbott KC, et al. De novo congestive heart failure after kidney transplantation: a common condition with poor prognostic implications. Am J Kidney Dis 2005;46:720.
[5] Go AS, Chertow GM, Fan D, et al. Chronic kidney disease and the risks of death, cardiovascular events, and hospitalization. N Engl J Med 2004;351:1296–305.
[6] Danovitch GM. The epidemic of cardiovascular disease in chronic renal disease: a challenge to the transplant physician. Graft 1999;2(Supp II):S108–12.
[7] Kasiske BL. Epidemiology of cardiovascular disease after renal transplantation. Transplantation 2001;72:S5–8.
[8] Brattstrom C, Wilczek HE, Tyden G, et al. Hypertriglyceridemia in renal transplant recipients treated with sirolimus. Transplant Proc 1998;30:3950.
[9] Steinman TI, Becker BN, Frost AE, et al. Guidelines for the referral and management of patients eligible for solid organ transplant. Transplantation 2001;71:1189–204.
[10] Kasiske BL, Ramos EL, Gaston RS, et al. The evaluation of renal transplant candidates: clinical practice guidelines. J Am Soc Nephrol 1996;6:1–28.
[11] Carey WD, Dumot JA, Pimentel RR, et al. The prevalence of coronary artery disease in liver transplant candidates over age 50. Transplantation 1995;59:859.
[12] Kaza AK, Dietz JF, Kern JA, et al. Coronary risk stratification in patients with end-stage lung disease. J Heart Lung Transplant 2002;21:334.
[13] Mangano DT, Layug EL, Wallace E, et al. Effect of atenolol on mortality and cardiovascular morbidity after noncardiac surgery: multicenter study of Perioperative Ischemia Research Group. N Engl J Med 1996;335:1713–25.

[14] Fishman JA, Rubin RH. Infection in organ transplant recipients. N Engl J Med 1998;338: 1741.

[15] Bratzler DW, Houck PM. Surgical Infection Prevention Writing Group. Antimicrobial prophylaxis for surgery: an advisory statement from the National Surgical Infection Prevention Project. Am J Surg 2005;189(4):395–404.

[16] Anstead GM. Steroids, retinoids and wound healing. Adv Wound Care 1998;11(6):277–85.

[17] Meadows EC, Prudden JF. A study of the influence of adrenal steroids on the strength of healing wounds; preliminary report. Surgery 1953;33(6):841–8.

[18] Dean PG, Lung WJ, Larson TS, et al. Wound-healing complications after kidney transplantation: a prospective, randomized comparison of sirolimus and tacrolimus. Transplantation 2004;77(10):1555–61.

[19] Bromberg JS, Alfrey EJ, Barker CF, et al. Adrenal suppression and steroid supplementation in renal transplant patients. Transplantation 1991;51:385–90.

[20] Glowniak JV, Loriaux DL. A double-blind study of perioperative steroid requirements in secondary adrenal insufficiency. Surgery 1997;121:123–9.

[21] Kehlet H, Binder C. Adrenocortical function and clinical course during and after surgery in unsupplemented glucocorticoid-treated patients. BMJ 1973;2:147–9.

[22] Bromberg JS, Baliga P, Cofer JB, et al. Stress steroids are not required for patients receiving a renal allograft and undergoing operation. J Am Coll Surg 1995;180(5):532–6.

[23] Salem M, Tainsh RE Jr, Bromberg J, et al. Perioperative glucocorticoid coverage. A reassessment 42 years after emergence of a problem. Ann Surg 1994;219:416–25.

[24] Irish A. Hypercoagulability in renal transplant recipients. Identifying patients at risk of renal allograft thrombosis and evaluating strategies for prevention. Am J Cardiovasc Drugs 2004; 4(3):139–49.

[25] Morrissey PE, Ramirez PJ, Gohh RY, et al. Management of thrombophilia in renal transplant patients. Am J Transplant 2002;2(9):872–6.

[26] Poge U, Gerhardt T, Palmedo H, et al. MDRD equations for estimation of GFR in renal transplant recipients. Am J Transplant 2005;5(6):1306–11.

[27] Burch PG, Stanski DR. Decreased protein binding and thiopental kinetics. Clin Pharmacol Ther 1982;32(2):212–7.

[28] Kurella M, Bennett WM, Chertow GM. Analgesia in patients with ESRD: a review of available evidence. Am J Kidney Dis 2003;42(2):217–28.

[29] Sear JW. Kidney transplants: induction and analgesic agents. Int Anesthesiol Clin 1995; 33(2):45–68.

[30] Ojo AO, Held PJ, Port FK, et al. Chronic renal failure after transplantation of a nonrenal organ. N Engl J Med 2003;349(10):931–40.

[31] Kostopangiotou G, Smyrniotis V, Arkadopoulos N, et al. Anesthetic and perioperative management of adult transplant recipients in nontransplant surgery. Anesth Analg 1999; 89(3):613–22.

[32] Wong F, Blendis LM. The patient with renal insufficiency. Liver Transplant Surg 1996;2(5): 35–43.

[33] Hoeper MM, Krowka MJ, Strassburg CP. Portopulmonary hypertension and hepatopulmonary syndrome. Lancet 2004;363(9419):1461–8.

[34] Eriksson JS, Soderman C, Ericzon BG, et al. Normalization of ventilation/perfusion relationships after liver transplantation in patients with decompensated cirrhosis: evidence for a hepatopulmonary syndrome. Hepatology 1990;12(6):1350–7.

[35] Krowka MJ. Hepatopulmonary syndrome: an evolving perspective in the era of liver transplantation. Hepatology 1990;12:1350–7.

[36] Csete M, Sipher MJ. Management of the transplant patient for nontransplant procedures. Adv Anesth 1994;11:407–31.

[37] Keegan MT, Plevak DJ. Preoperative assessment of the patient with liver disease. Am J Gastroenterol 2005;100(9):2116–27.

[38] Gelb AW, Sharpe MD. Organ transplantation: anesthetic considerations for the previously transplanted patient. In: Benumof JL, editor. Anesthesiology clinics of North America. Philadelphia (PA): WB Saunders; 1994. p. 827–43.

[39] Trulock EP, Edwards LB, Taylor DO, et al. Registry of the International Society for Heart and Lung Transplantation: twenty-second official adult lung and heart-lung transplant report—2005. J Heart Lung Transplant 2005;24(8):956–67.

[40] Trachiotis GD, Knight SR, Hann M, et al. Respiratory responses to $CO_2$ rebreathing in lung transplant recipients. Ann Thorac Surg 1994;58:1709–17.

[41] Levy RD, Ernst P, Levine SM, et al. Exercise performance after lung transplantation. J Heart Lung Transplant 1993;12:27–33.

[42] Arcasoy SM, Kotloff RM. Lung transplantation. N Engl J Med 1999;340:1080–91.

[43] Wekerle T, Klepetko W, Wisser W, et al. Incidence and outcome of major non-pulmonary surgical procedures in lung transplant recipients. Eur J Cardiothorac Surg 1997;12:718–23.

[44] Sharpe MD. Anaesthesia and the transplanted patient. Can J Anaesth 1996;43(5 Pt 2):R89–98.

[45] Higenbottam T, Jackson P, Woolman R, et al. The cough response to ultrasonically nebulized distilled water in heart–lung transplantation patients. Am Rev Respir Dis 1989;140:58–61.

[46] Herve P, Silbert J, Cerrina G, et al. Impairment of bronchial mucociliary clearance in long-term survivors of heart/lung and double-lung transplantation. The Paris-Sud Lung Transplant Group. Chest 1993;103(1):59–63.

[47] Trulock EP. State of the art lung transplantation. Am J Respir Crit Care Med 1997;155: 789–818.

[48] Ruggiero R, Muz J, Fietsem R Jr, et al. Reestablishment of lymphatic drainage after canine lung transplantation. J Thorac Cardiovasc Surg 1993;106(1):167–71.

[49] Haddow GR, Brock-Utne JG. A non-thoracic operation for a patient with single lung transplantation. Acta Anaesthesiol Scan 1999;43(9):960–3.

[50] Gavazzeni V, Iapichino G, Mascheroni D, et al. Prolonged independent lung respiratory treatment after single lung transplantation in pulmonary emphysema. Chest 1993;103(1): 96–100.

[51] Taylor DO, Edwards LB, Boucek MM, et al. Registry of the International Society for Heart and Lung Transplantation: twenty-second official adult heart transplant report—2005. J Heart Lung Transplant 2005;24(8):945–55.

[52] Brann WM, Bennet LE, Keck BM, et al. Morbidity, functional status, and immunosuppressive therapy after heart transplantation: an analysis of the joint International Society for Heart and Lung Transplantation/United Network for Organ Sharing Thoracic Registry. J Heart Lung Transplant 1998;17(4):374–82.

[53] Smith ML, Ellenbogen KA, Eckberg DL, et al. Subnormal parasympathetic activity after cardiac transplantation. Am J Cardiol 1990;66:1243–6.

[54] Younis L, Melin J, Schoevaerdts J, et al. Left ventricular systolic function and diastolic filling at rest and during upright exercise after orthotopic heart transplantation: comparison with young and aged normal subjects. J Heart Transplant 1990;9(6):683–92.

[55] von Scheidt W, Zeigler U, Kemkes BM, et al. Heart transplantation: hemodynamics over a five-year period. J Heart Lung Transplant 1991;10(3):342–50.

[56] Jensen M, Olivari M, Walt MT, et al. Frequency and significance of right bundle branch block after cardiac transplantation. Am J Cardiol 1994;73(13):1009–11.

[57] Leonelli F, Pacifico A, Young J. Frequency and significance of conduction defects early after orthotopic heart transplantation. Am J Cardiol 1994;73:175–9.

[58] Miller L. Long-term complications of cardiac transplantation. Prog Cardiovasc Dis 1991;33: 229–82.

[59] Behrendt D, Ganz P, Fang JC. Cardiac allograft vasculopathy. Curr Opin Cardiol 2000;15: 422–9.

[60] Bristow MR. The surgically denervated, transplanted, human heart. Circulation 1990;82: 658–60.

[61] Cheng DC, Ong DD. Anesthesia for non-cardiac surgery in heart-transplanted patients. Can J Anaesth 1993;40:981–6.

[62] Manske CL, Wilson RF, Wang Y, et al. Atherosclerotic vascular complications in diabetic transplant candidates. Am J Kidney Dis 1997;29:601–7.

[63] Kennedy WR, Navarro X, Goetz FC, et al. Effects of pancreatic transplantation on diabetic neuropathy. N Engl J Med 1990;322(15):1031–7.

[64] Paty BW, Lanz K, Kendall DM, et al. Restored hypoglycemic counterregulation is stable in successful pancreas transplant recipients for up to 19 years after transplantation. Transplantation 2001;72(6):1103–7.

[65] Del Pizzo JJ, Jacobs SC, Bartlet ST, et al. Urologic complications of bladder-drained pancreatic allografts. Br J Urol 1998;81:543–7.

SURGICAL
CLINICS OF
NORTH AMERICA

Surg Clin N Am 86 (2006) 1167–1183

# Perioperative Management of Immunosuppression

Sonia Lin, PharmD[a],*, Christopher J. Cosgrove, MD[b]

[a]Department of Pharmacy Practice, College of Pharmacy, University of Rhode Island,
144 Fogarty Hall, Kingston, RI 02881, USA
[b]Division of Nephrology, Transplant Section, Rhode Island Hospital,
593 Eddy Street, PAC 921, Providence, RI 02903, USA

Immunosuppressive therapy for the prevention of rejection in solid-organ transplantation has made notable progress since the first successful nontwin kidney transplantation was performed in 1959. Early attempts with organ transplantation using total-body irradiation resulted in overimmunosuppression and overwhelming infections. Promising results with an antineoplastic agent, 6-mercaptopurine, in animal studies led to the introduction of its prodrug, azathioprine (AZA), in 1962. The application of AZA in combination with corticosteroids resulted in 1-year graft survival rates of 40% to 50%; this was considered revolutionary in clinical transplantation. Until that time, with hemodialysis in its earliest stages, survival with renal failure was exceedingly rare. Several more potent immunosuppressive agents have become available since then, leading to the successful transplantation of more than 25,000 organs annually in the United States, including nonrenal solid-organ transplants such as liver, pancreas, heart, and lung [1]. At 1 year, graft and patient survival rates of up to 95% and 98% can be achieved, respectively, with living donors, and 80% and 90% of patients are supported by a functioning deceased donor allograft, depending on the organ.

Current immunosuppressive regimens typically consist of two phases: induction phase and maintenance therapy. The various agents that are used in these two phases of immunosuppression will be reviewed in this article. The similarities and differences between the agents within each class, with respect to efficacy and tolerability, will also be discussed.

---

* Corresponding author.
E-mail address: SLin@uri.edu (S. Lin).

doi:10.1016/j.suc.2006.06.013
*surgical.theclinics.com*

**Induction therapy in solid-organ transplantation**

The greatest risk of rejection of a transplanted organ occurs in the immediate period (weeks to months) after implantation. Thereafter, the risk of rejection is intermediate in the first year after placement and low, but omnipresent for the life of the transplanted organ. As such, induction strategies aim to reduce early acute rejection episodes and prolong long-term allograft survival. Most regimens for induction therapy also attempt to minimize the complications of maintenance immunosuppression. There are no standardized induction regimens, but most transplant centers use one of two basic strategies: (1) the use of high doses of conventional immunosuppressive agents, or (2) the use of polyclonal or monoclonal antibodies directed against T-cell antigens. This section discusses the agents used in the latter strategy.

The decision to use induction therapy with either polyclonal or monoclonal antibodies is dependent upon several factors including:

1. The organ transplanted: use of antibody induction is common in heart, lung, and kidney transplantation, occasional in liver transplantation, and almost universal with pancreas transplantation.
2. The immunologic risk of the recipient: induction agents are more commonly used in high-risk patients such as those of African decent, repeat (second or greater) transplants, and those patients with preformed anti-human leukocyte antigen (HLA) antibodies.
3. Planned minimization of maintenance immunosuppression, usually involving steroids or calcineurin inhibitors (cyclosporine and tacrolimus).

*Polyclonal antibodies*

There are two polyclonal agents in use today for induction therapy: horse antithymocyte globulin (ATGAM; Pharmacia-UpJohn, Kalamazoo, Michigan) and rabbit antithymocyte globulin (rATG; Thymoglobulin, Genzyme, Cambridge, Massachusetts). ATGAM is derived from horse sera immunized against human lymphocytes and Thymoglobulin from the sera of immunized rabbit. Both of these agents contain antibodies against a wide variety of T-cell surface antigens and act to deplete CD3-positive cells in the recipient. The depletion of lymphocytes occurs through a variety of mechanisms including complement-mediated and Fc-dependent opsonization and lysis [2]. Rabbit-ATG has become the polyclonal agent of choice, both for improved allograft survival as well as an observed decrease in delayed graft function (DGF) [3]. The original licensing for rATG was based on its efficacy for the treatment of acute rejection. The more frequent off-label use of the agent for immunosuppression induction follows from previous experience with polyclonal antibodies and the published experience within the transplant community. Both polyclonal agents have been used for the treatment of rejection, with rATG demonstrating superiority in both reversal of rejection, as well as preventing recurrent rejection [4,5]. Some of this observed benefit might be related to the specific processing that makes rATG a more uniform product (less batch-to-batch variability), resulting in a more consistent clinical effect. Indeed, both the degree of lymphocyte depletion and the response to therapy are more predictable with the rATG product.

The use of polyclonal antibodies is associated with a "first-dose reaction," manifesting as fevers and chills. This syndrome results from the release of inflammatory cytokines from lymphocytes as a consequence of activation, lysis, or destruction. Most centers administer steroids and often a combination of acetaminophen, antihistamines, pentoxifylline, and other agents to abrogate this response. Severe cases may be associated with capillary leak syndrome and pulmonary edema. Other reactions include anemia, thrombocytopenia, rash, pruritis, serum sickness, and rarely, anaphylaxis. The occurrence of adverse events is, in part, related to the timing and rate of administration, with intraoperative administration and slow infusion being less likely to produce severe first dose reactions.

*Monoclonal antibodies*

The oldest monoclonal antibody is Muromonab-CD3 (OKT-3, Orthoclone; Ortho Biotech, Bridgewater, New Jersey), which has been in use since 1986. OKT-3 is a murine IgG2 monoclonal antibody targeting the CD3 complex on T-lymphocytes, and like the polyclonal antibodies, induces a rapid depletion of T-lymphocytes [6]. OKT-3 has been used for both induction therapy and treatment of steroid resistant rejection. It is, however, associated with the release of several pro-inflammatory cytokines, and can cause the cytokine release syndrome, manifesting as fever, chills, headache, gastrointestinal symptoms, and most significantly, noncardiogenic pulmonary edema and acute respiratory distress syndrome [7]. These symptoms are ameliorated through premedication with steroids and antihistamines. OKT-3 also induces production of human antimouse antibodies (HAMA, antibodies generated against the agent) in nearly 50% of patients who undergo therapy with it, which may preclude future use [8].

Daclizumab (Zenapax; Roche Laboratories, Nutley, New Jersey) and basiliximab (Simulect; Novartis Pharmaceuticals, Inc, East Hanover, New Jersey) are monoclonal antibodies that do not cause depletion of T-cell populations but rather block IL-2 mediated T-cell activation, preventing rejection. Daclizumab is a humanized antibody, which combines a mouse hypervariable region with human IgG, and basiliximab is a chimeric antibody that combines mouse antigen-binding variable regions with human IgG constant regions. Both anti-IL2 receptor antibodies appear to have equal efficacy in clinical trials, reducing the incidence of acute rejection by 33% to 50% when added to maintenance immunosuppression. The two agents have not been compared against one another in direct studies

[9–12]. A significant difference occurs in the dosage administration schedule as daclizumab is dosed at the time of transplant with four additional doses at 2-week intervals, whereas basiliximab is dosed on the day of surgery and the fourth postoperative day. Both of these agents are associated with minimal side effects compared with the other agents. They have no role in the treatment of acute rejection. Of interest is the observation that basiliximab, a drug with minimal side effects and presumably less "potent" than polyclonal antibodies, resulted in similar incidence of acute rejection compared with rATG in low-risk kidney transplant recipients [13].

Alemtuzumab (Campath-1H; Genzyme Oncology, Cambridge, Massachusetts) is the newest molecule to be used for induction therapy in solid-organ transplantation. The monoclonal antibody was developed for the treatment of chronic lymphocytic leukemia, with reports of full remissions. Alemtuzumab is specific for the common lymphocyte and monocyte antigen CD52. Its administration temporarily depletes mature lymphocytes and some monocytes without altering neutrophils or hematopoietic stem cells. The agent has a profound and long-lasting effect on the depletion of white blood cells [14].

Alemtuzumab has been used for induction in kidney, liver, heart, lung, and pancreas transplantation. Intravenous regimens of alemtuzumab, consisting of either a single 30 mg dose or two 20 mg doses, when used in conjunction with standard maintenance immunosuppressive agents, resulted in comparable rates of acute rejection, and patient and graft survival rates that are seen using induction therapy with rATG or anti-IL2 receptor antagonists [15–18]. Alemtuzumab also facilitates steroid-free immunosuppression in more than 80% of patients in conjunction with lower doses of other immunosuppressive agents such as calcineurin inhibitors [15–20]. Infusion-related adverse reactions have been associated with intravenous alemtuzumab administration, and can range from moderate symptoms such as fevers, chills, rigors, hypotension, and bronchospasm, to more life-threatening reactions such as arrhythmias, myocardial infarction, and respiratory or cardiac arrest. These adverse reactions can be avoided by premedicating with corticosteroids, acetaminophen, and diphenhydramine [21]. Alemtuzumab induction appears promising in the era of maintenance immunosuppression minimization; however, its potent effects on leukocyte depletion and the development of infection and malignancy requires evaluation in long-term controlled studies.

## Maintenance immunosuppression

Standard maintenance immunosuppression regimens generally consist of a triple-drug combination, comprised of agents that act simultaneously at different levels of the immune cascade. Corticosteroids, calcineurin inhibitors, antiproliferatives, and mTOR inhibitors are the available immunosuppressive drug classes in use today. The most common regimen incorporates a calcineurin inhibitor, an antiproliferative agent, and corticosteroids. Variations of this regimen are driven by the organ recipient's immunologic risk for rejection, the immunogenicity of the allograft (lung > heart > kidney > liver) and medication-related toxicities that develop [22]. As a result, it is not uncommon for low-risk recipients and recipients of liver transplants to be on a single or two-drug regimen with stable allograft function.

## Corticosteroids

Corticosteroids have been a key component of most maintenance immunosuppressive protocols across all solid organ transplants since the 1960s [1]. The mechanism of immunosuppressive action is incompletely understood, but it is known that corticosteroids block T- and B-cell activation via intracellular inhibition of interleukin (IL) and cytokine gene transcription [23]. Corticosteroids also induce a general lymphopenia by redirecting lymphocytes from the periphery to the lymphoid tissue and release of anti-inflammatory mediators leading to leukocytosis, elevated glucose concentrations, and central antipyretic effects [24].

Corticosteroid regimens vary widely, typically with higher doses initially and then tapered over a period of 3 to 6 months to maintenance doses equivalent to prednisone 5 to 10 mg, which is further tapered slowly over time. Intravenous high-dose corticosteroids are also commonly used for the treatment of acute rejection across all solid-organ transplants [1]. The main oral and intravenous corticosteroid agents used in practice are prednisone and methylprednisolone, respectively. The use of prednisolone is preferred in patients with hepatic insufficiency who cannot metabolize prednisone to its active counterpart. Dexamethasone has also been used in place of methylprednisolone with equal efficacy [25]. The equipotent doses and relative anti-inflammatory and mineralocorticoid potencies of these agents are summarized in Table 1 [26].

Table 1
Comparison of commonly used corticosteroids in solid organ transplantation

| Corticosteroid | Route of administration | Anti-inflammatory potency | Equivalent dose (mg) | Mineralocorticoid activity | Duration of action (hours) |
|---|---|---|---|---|---|
| Hydrocortisone | IV, PO | 1 | 20 | 1 | 8–12 |
| Prednisone | PO | 4 | 5 | 0.8 | 24 |
| Prednisolone | PO | 4 | 5 | 0.8 | 24 |
| Methlyprednisolone | IV | 5 | 4 | 0.5 | 36 |
| Dexamethasone | IV, PO | 25 | 0.75 | 0 | 72 |

*Adapted from* Schimmer BP, Parker KL. Adrenocorticotropic hormone; adrenocortical steroids and their synthetic analogs; inhibitors of the synthesis and actions of adrenocortical hormones. In: Brunton LL, editor, Goodman & Gilman's The pharmacologic basis of therapeutics. 11th edition. New York: McGraw-Hill Medical Publishing Division, 2006. p. 1587–612.

Corticosteroids are associated with numerous well-known adverse effects including hypertension (HTN), hyperlipidemia, posttransplant diabetes mellitus (PTDM), osteoporosis, and cataracts [27]. Of major concern, HTN, lipid abnormalities, and diabetes are all risk factors that are associated with cardiovascular disease (CVD). Concomitant use with other immunosuppressive agents can exacerbate these abnormalities [28]. There is a trend toward adopting corticosteroid minimization protocols in an effort to avoid these long-term adverse effects. Preventative strategies established in the general population may be applied to the transplant population when indicated [29]. Adrenal suppression can also occur as a long-term consequence of corticosteroid therapy and manifest as overt adrenal insufficiency with hypotension under stressful conditions such as general anesthesia and surgery. Recommendations for steroid replacement vary widely for transplant patients requiring nontransplant surgery. Simply continuing baseline doses of corticosteroids is sufficient in the majority of cases [30]. This may be particularly true as smaller doses of steroids become more widely adopted in clinical practice. Despite this experience and the absence of controlled studies that demonstrate a requirement for stress-dose steroids in this circumstance, most authors recommend a perioperative increase in steroids, typically hydrocortisone, with a rapid return to baseline doses based on the extent of the surgery and recovery [31].

## Calcineurin inhibitors

Calcineurin inhibitors have been an integral part of immunosuppressive therapy for transplantation since the 1980s, and are currently used in the vast majority of transplant recipients upon discharge from the hospital after the transplant procedure [1]. Cyclosporine (CsA) and tacrolimus inhibit IL-2 mediated T-cell activation and lymphocyte proliferation through binding with their respective immunophilin proteins, cyclophilin and FK-binding protein [32,33]. This specific drug–immunophilin complex binds with and inhibits calcineurin, preventing transit of the transcription factor, nuclear factor of activated T cells, to the DNA promoter region thereby inhibiting IL-2 synthesis.

CsA was initially released as an oil-based oral formulation (Sandimmune; Novartis Pharmaceuticals, East Hanover, New Jersey), which was largely dependent on the extent of solubilization in bile, and thus had an erratic absorption profile. The microemulsion formulation (Neoral; Novartis Pharmaceuticals, East Hanover, New Jersey), with more predictable pharmacokinetics, has largely replaced the use of Sandimmune [32]. Generic formulations of CsA are also currently available, and although some of these products are rated as therapeutically equivalent (AB-rated) by the Food and Drug Administration, consistent use of one oral formulation is preferred versus routine switching between products. Further discussion of CsA in this review will refer to the microemulsion formulation. CsA can also be administered as an intermittent intravenous infusion at one-third of the maintenance oral dose [34]. Tacrolimus is available for administration orally or intravenously as well; intravenous tacrolimus is administered as a 24-hour infusion versus an intermittent infusion, also at approximately one-third of the oral dose [35].

CsA and tacrolimus are both effective in reducing the incidence of acute rejection after transplantation [36,37]; however, improved outcomes have been observed with tacrolimus when used in blacks [38,39] and those with DGF [38]. The use of calcineurin inhibitors allows safe withdrawal of corticosteroid therapy in liver transplant recipients without increased risk for rejection [40]. Tacrolimus-based regimens also facilitate corticosteroid withdrawal and avoidance in kidney transplantation, particularly when used in conjunction with induction agents [41–43].

Routine therapeutic drug monitoring (TDM) is required for calcineurin inhibitors due to their narrow therapeutic index for efficacy and toxicity. Peak 2-hour (C2) CsA levels are better correlated with overall drug exposure than CsA trough (C0) levels; however, it is often logistically difficult to obtain these levels accurately; thus, C0 levels are more frequently used [32,34]. Target C0 and C2 levels range from 150 to 400 ng/mL and 800 to 2000 ng/mL, respectively. Tacrolimus target whole-blood C0 levels are generally 5 to 20 ng/mL [44]. Higher doses are usually required in black patients due to pharmacogenomic differences in p-glycoprotein and CYP450 enzyme expression [45,46]. Doses and target levels for both drugs vary, and are adjusted depending on the transplant type and the amount of time that has lapsed posttransplant.

The pharmacokinetic profiles of these calcineurin inhibitors are very similar. Both drugs undergo extensive first pass effect via p-glycoprotein and intestinal and hepatic CYP450 3A enzymes after oral administration. Both drugs are extensively metabolized in the liver by the same enzyme system. Metabolites are primarily eliminated in the bile, with a small percentage of the dose being excreted unchanged in the urine [32,44]. Calcineurin inhibitors have the potential for many drug–drug interactions due to their reliance on the CYP540 enzyme system for drug clearance. Concomitant use of drugs that induce or inhibit CYP450 enzymes should be used with caution. The most common class of agents includes antimicrobial agents such as azoles and macrolides. More vigilant TDM of CsA or tacrolimus drug levels is required; in some cases, dose adjustment should be made in addition, concurrent with commencing antimicrobial therapy [47]. Changes in gut motility can also affect the extent of drug absorption, and hence, overall drug exposure. One might expect reduced drug absorption due to decreased gut transit time as a result of diarrhea. Paradoxically, increases in tacrolimus trough concentrations requiring dose reduction have been observed in patients with persistent diarrhea. This is likely a result of decreased intestinal p-glycoprotein activity due to diarrhea-induced mucosal damage [48].

The most well-known adverse effect of calcineurin inhibitors is nephrotoxicity. Chronic allograft nephropathy is a major cause of graft failure in kidney transplant recipients and calcineurin inhibitor-induced nephrotoxicity is a contributing factor [49]. Calcineurin inhibitor-induced renal toxicity has also been reported in about 10% to 20% of nonrenal transplant recipients [50]. Diabetes mellitus is another well-known adverse effect of calcineurin inhibitors and is a significant risk factor for CVD [51]. The incidence of nephrotoxicity and PTDM is similar between the two agents, although there are trends toward improved renal function with tacrolimus and improved glucose control with CsA [38,52]. Rates of PTDM of less than 5% have been reported for CsA and with regimens targeting lower tacrolimus trough levels when used in conjunction with minimal corticosteroid doses. Risk factors for developing PTDM include increased age, black ethnicity, hepatitis C virus, and concomitant administration of high-dose corticosteroids [53].

Other common adverse effects of calcineurin inhibitors include neurotoxicity, cardiovascular disturbances, and cosmetic effects [33]. Neurotoxic effects are more frequently associated with tacrolimus therapy, and can range from mild symptoms such as headache and tremor to more severe effects such as seizures, delirium, and coma. Alopecia and electrolyte disturbances, such as hyperkalemia and hypomagnesemia, are also more common with tacrolimus. Conversely, CsA is associated with a greater incidence of cardiovascular effects, such as hypertension and hyperlipidemia, and cosmetic effects, such as gingival hyperplasia and hirsutism [32,44]. Perhaps more so than the modest clinical improvements demonstrated for tacrolimus, these CsA-induced adverse effects on blood lipids and cosmesis resulted in tacrolimus gaining over 80% of the market in solid-organ transplantation.

## Antiproliferatives

AZA, an inhibitor of purine nucleotide synthesis, was the first immunosuppressive agent to be used with significant success in clinical transplantation. AZA is metabolized via the enzymes thiopurine S-methyltransferase and xanthine oxidase to inactive metabolites, which are subsequently excreted in the urine [54]. Concomitant use of allopurinol in patients with gout should be approached with caution due to its inhibitory effect on xanthine oxidase. Doses of AZA should be reduced by at least two-thirds of the usual dose to avoid AZA-related toxicity [55]. Bone marrow suppression is a major dose-related adverse effect in almost 50% of patients. Gastrointestinal (GI) adverse effects such as nausea and vomiting, hepatitis, cholestasis, and rarely pancreatitis, can also occur with AZA therapy [54].

With the introduction of mycophenolate mofetil (MMF) in 1995, a noticeable shift has occurred with the declining use of AZA and a corresponding increase in MMF use over the last 10 years. MMF has largely replaced AZA as the antiproliferative agent in maintenance immunosuppression across the majority of solid-organ transplants [1]. MMF is the ester prodrug of mycophenolic acid (MPA), a potent inhibitor of inosine monophosphate dehydrogenase (IMDPH). IMDPH is an enzyme expressed in T- and B-lymphocytes, and is required for de novo guanosine synthesis; inhibition of IMDPH results in the suppression of DNA synthesis and lymphocyte proliferation [56]. The usual starting dose is 2 g/d administered orally or intravenously in two divided doses [57]. Higher doses of 3 g/d may be required in black recipients [58].

After oral administration, MMF is rapidly hydrolyzed to its active metabolite MPA via the first pass effect. MPA is then metabolized mainly to its inactive glucuronide metabolite, MPAG, through the enzyme UDP-glucuronyltransferase (UDPGT) and excreted through the urine. MPAG also undergoes enterohepatic recirculation, whereby it is excreted in the bile, converted back to MPA by gut flora, specifically Gram-negative anaerobes, and is reabsorbed back into the circulation [57]. Both MPA and MPAG are bound to serum albumin; accumulation of MPAG can result in competition for albumin binding sites with MPA [59]. Finally, renal impairment results in MPAG accumulation, leading to displacement of MPA from albumin binding sites; uremia also has the same effect [60]. This may result in an increased risk of adverse effects in kidney transplant patients with delayed or slow graft function and calcineurin inhibitor-induced or other forms of renal dysfunction. Major complaints associated with MMF therapy are gastrointestinal adverse effects, such as nausea and diarrhea [61], and hematologic toxicities such as leukopenia and anemia [57]. An increased incidence of tissue invasive cytomegalovirus disease, particularly gastrointestinal, is also associated with MMF doses of greater than 2 g/d [62].

Enteric-coated mycophenolate sodium (Myfortic, EC-MPS) is a delayed-release formulation of MPA that was designed to reduce upper GI toxicity. It has similar efficacy and toxicity as MMF in de novo kidney transplant patients [63]. Administration of 720 mg doses resulted in similar MPA exposure as MMF doses of 1000 mg [64]. Patients who are intolerant of MMF due to GI adverse effects may be able to continue with therapy using EC-MPS; however, this potential benefit is controversial as GI adverse events correlate with systemic drug levels rather than local exposure [65]. To date, randomized trials of EC-MPS compared with MMF have demonstrated similar efficacy, and no clinically significant reduction in side effects.

Routine TDM is not required with antiproliferative therapy; however, its clinical value in MMF therapy is being explored [66]. MPA trough levels have been shown to predict acute rejection episodes and MMF-related toxicity such as diarrhea, leukopenia, anemia, and viral infections in kidney transplantation [67]. However, threshold values may vary depending on the type of organ transplant, and further study is required before TDM can be routinely advocated for MMF.

The potential for many drug–drug interactions to affect the pharmacokinetics of MPA exists, particularly when MMF is coadministered with other immunosuppressive agents [68]. Higher MPA trough levels are achieved in patients receiving tacrolimus versus CsA, necessitating the use of lower MMF doses [69,70]. This primarily occurs due to the inhibitory effect of CsA on MPAG biliary excretion, thus interrupting enterohepatic circulation [71,72]. However, it has also been demonstrated that tacrolimus has an inhibitory effect on the UDPGT enzyme, leading to elevations in MPA levels due to decreased glucuronidation to MPAG [73]. Adverse effects or acute rejection may be precipitated, and should be considered when patients are switching from CsA to tacrolimus or vice versa, respectively. Corticosteroids are known inducers of drug-metabolizing enzymes, such as UDPGT; thus, withdrawal or avoidance can also result in relatively higher MPA levels [74]. Other drugs that have been shown to affect the pharmacokinetics of MPA include metronidazole, norfloxacin, antacids, and cholestyramine, all of which interfere with enterohepatic recirculation, reducing the overall exposure of MPA and MPAG. Concurrent administration of metronidazole and norfloxacin inhibit bacterial deglucuronidation of MPAG to MPA. Although interactions with other antibiotics have not been reported, patients should be carefully observed for signs of acute rejection upon initiation of other antibiotic therapy with activity against Gram-negative organisms [75]. The interaction with antacids and cholestyramine is physicochemical in nature; they bind to MMF or MPA, respectively, leading to reduced absorption [59]. Thus, TDM of MPA may be important in optimizing MMF therapy in transplant patients, given the continuous fine tuning of immunosuppressive regimens based on individual patients' therapeutic response and tolerance to adverse drug effects, as well as the trend toward minimization of immunosuppression as patient and graft survival increases.

## mTOR inhibitors

Sirolimus (Rapamune; Wyeth Pharmaceuticals, Madison, New Jersey) was introduced into the armamentarium of immunosuppressive agents in 2000. Sirolimus complexes with mTOR via the FK-binding protein, resulting in arrest of the G1 to S phase of the cell cycle in various cell types. Sirolimus is effective when used in combination with calcineurin inhibitors or antiproliferative agents in all solid-organ transplants, and allows lower calcineurin inhibitor doses to be used to minimize the risk for nephrotoxicity. Patients exhibiting signs of chronic allograft dysfunction or calcineurin inhibitor-induced nephrotoxicity may also benefit from a switch to a sirolimus-based regimen as early as 3 months posttransplantation [76–79]. Incorporation of sirolimus into current immunosuppressive regimens may be advantageous in that it demonstrates antineoplastic properties; the risk of de novo malignancy and a nonskin de novo solid cancer was reduced by more than 50% in association with mTOR inhibitor therapy [80,81]. However, its use in liver and lung recipients immediately posttransplant is limited by the risk of hepatic artery thrombosis and airway anastomotic dehiscence, respectively [82–84]. In addition, risk of thrombotic microangiopathy is associated with concomitant use of sirolimus and CsA in kidney and kidney–pancreas recipients [85].

Sirolimus is available in tablet and liquid formulations, but is not available as an injectable. Conversion between the tablet and liquid formulations can be made on a milligram-per-milligram basis based on pharmacokinetic studies demonstrating similar overall drug exposure [86]. The absolute bioavailability is low at about 15%, and is further reduced if the dose is administered with a high fat meal. Sirolimus is metabolized via the CYP450 3A enzyme system and p-glycoprotein; metabolites are primarily eliminated in the feces with minimal excretion in the urine [87]. Inhibitors or inducers of these two metabolic pathways that affect calcineurin inhibitors will likely also affect sirolimus. Lower CsA doses are required to maintain similar trough levels when administered with sirolimus. This is likely due to an interaction between sirolimus and CsA at the CYP450 and p-glycoprotein level.

Sirolimus has a long terminal half-life of 62 hours, which allows once-daily administration. Upon initiation of therapy, a loading dose of three times the maintenance dose is required to achieve steady-state concentrations more rapidly. Trough whole-blood sirolimus levels of less than 5 ng/ml and greater than 15 ng/ml are associated with the occurrence of acute rejection episodes and a greater incidence of adverse effects, respectively. TDM of trough whole-blood levels should occur no more often than weekly after initiation of therapy or dose changes [86,87].

The most common adverse effects observed with sirolimus include thrombocytopenia, leukopenia, anemia, hypertriglyceridemia, hypercholesterolemia, diarrhea, and acne/mouth ulcers. These dose-dependent toxicities are either self-limiting or can be managed with dose reductions [88]. Other less common, but important adverse effects occurs as a result of the antiproliferative properties of sirolimus. Despite its lack of nephrotoxicity, sirolimus may delay recovery after renal injury increasing the risk of DGF, as well as prolonging recovery from DGF [89]. Sirolimus is associated with an increased frequency of lymphoceles, nonlymphocele perinephric fluid collections, peripheral edema, and wound complications, particularly in the presence of other risk factors such as obesity, DM, infection, rejection, and increased age [90]. Finally, interstitial alveolar pneumonitis is a rare and potentially fatal complication of sirolimus therapy. Withdrawal of therapy results in symptomatic improvement within a few days to weeks with complete radiologic resolution within 3 to 10 months [91–94].

## Emerging immunosuppressive agents

A number of new immunosuppressive agents are in the late stages of development and are entering clinical trials. FTY720 is a synthetic analog of Myriocin, which affects T-cell trafficking. Its mechanism of action involves the sequestration of lymphocytes in lymphoid organs, minimizing the number of circulating lymphocytes. It has been associated with a reduction of acute rejection when used in combination with CsA and steroids [95]. An initial phase III trial in kidney transplant recipients failed to demonstrate equivalence with standard immunosuppression; however, the drug has shown promising therapeutic results in multiple sclerosis. LEA29Y is a receptor fusion protein that blocks T-cell activation by binding to CD80 and CD86. It is derived from a molecule, which has been shown to induce tolerance in rodent and primate models [96]. A great deal of promise exists for costimulatory blockade as a treatment strategy in transplantation based on several animal experiments, which demonstrated robust effects in the maintenance of allografts. LEA29Y is currently in phase II trials, and has been associated with less renal toxicity and less dyslipidemia. Leflunomide, an agent that inhibits de novo pyrimidine biosynthesis through the inhibition of the enzyme dihydroorotate dehydrogenase, is used off-label in transplantation as an antiproliferative agent [97]. Leflunomide has some antiviral properties, particularly against BK virus, creating a unique niche for this agent in kidney transplantation [97,98]. FK778 is a synthetic compound derived from the active metabolite of leflunomide. In preclinical trials, it appears to prevent the development of graft vasculopathy, which is typically seen in chronic rejection [99].

## Summary

Immunosuppressive therapy for solid-organ transplantation has evolved dramatically; current regimens yield excellent 1-year patient and graft survival rates. Despite the efficacy of currently available agents, there is the potential for significant drug interactions and adverse effects that may interfere with patient management for nontransplant surgical procedures. Awareness of the nuances between agents will allow general surgeons to manage the complications of immunosuppression without compromising efficacy. Future immunosuppressive agents will hopefully facilitate further individualization of drug therapy based on patient response and tolerability, leading to improved long-term outcome.

## References

[1] 2004 Annual Report of the US Organ Procurement and Transplantation Network and the Scientific Registry of Transplant Recipients: Transplant Data 1994–2003. Department of Health and Human Services, Health Resources and Services Administration, Healthcare Systems Bureau, Division of Transplantation, Rockville, MD; United Network for Organ Sharing, Richmond, VA; University Renal Research and Education Association, Ann Arbor, MI.

[2] Taniguchi Y, Frickhofen N, Raghavachar A, et al. Antilymphocyte immunoglobulins stimulate peripheral blood lymphocytes to proliferate and release lymphokines. Eur J Hematol 1990;44(4):244–51.

[3] Goggins WC, Pascual MA, Powelson JA, et al. A prospective, randomized, clinical trial of intraoperative versus postoperative Thymoglobulin in adult cadaveric renal transplant recipients. Transplantation 2003;76:798–802.

[4] Gaber AO, First K, Tesi RJ, et al. Results of the double-blind, randomized, multicenter, phase III clinical trial of Thymoglobulin versus Atgam in the treatment of acute graft rejection episodes after renal transplantation. Transplantation 1998;66:29.

[5] Brennan DC, Flavin K, Lowell JA, et al. A randomized double-blinded comparison of Thymoglobulin versus Atgam for induction immunosuppressive therapy in adult renal transplant recipients. Transplantation 1999;67:1011.

[6] Hong JC, Kahan BD. Immunosuppressive agents in organ transplantation: past, present, and future. Semin Nephrol 2000;20(2):108–25.

[7] Sgro C. Side effects of a monoclonal antibody, muromonab CD3/orthoclone OKT3: bibliographic review. Toxicology 1995;105:23–9.

[8] Kimball JA, Norman DJ, Shield CF, et al. The OKT3 antibody response study: a multicenter study of human anti-mouse antibody (HAMA) production following OKT3 use in solid organ transplantation. Transpl Immunol 1995;3:212–21.

[9] Vincenti F, Kirkman R, Light S, et al. Interleukin-2-receptor blockade with daclizumab to prevent acute rejection in renal transplantation. N Engl J Med 1998;338:161–5.

[10] Nashan B, Light S, Hardie IR, et al. Reduction of acute renal allograft rejection by daclizumab. Daclizumab Double Therapy Study Group. Transplantation 1999;67:110–5.

[11] Nashan B, Moore R, Amlot P, et al. Randomized trial of basiliximab versus placebo for control of acute cellular rejection in renal allograft recipients. CHIB 201 International Study Group. Lancet 1997;350(9086):1193–8.

[12] Kahan BD, Rajagopalan PR, Hall M. Reduction of the occurrence of acute cellular rejection among renal allograft recipients treated with basiliximab, a chimeric anti-interleuken-2-receptor monoclonal antibody. United States Simulect Renal Study Group. Transplantation 1999;67(2):276–84.

[13] Sollinger H, Kaplan B, Pescovitz MD, et al. Basiliximab versus antithymocyte globulin for prevention of acute renal allograft rejection. Transplantation 2001;72(12):1915–9.

[14] Taylor AL, Watson CJE, Bradley JA. Immunosuppressive agents in solid organ transplantation: mechanisms of action and therapeutic efficacy. Crit Rev Oncol Hemeatol 2005;56:23–46.

[15] Kaufman DB, Leventhal JR, Axelrod D, et al. Alemtuzumab induction and prednisone-free maintenance immunotherapy in kidney transplantation: comparison with basiliximab induction – long-term results. Am J Transplant 2005;5(10):2539–48.

[16] Cianco G, Burke GW, Gaynor JJ, et al. A randomized trial of three renal transplant induction antibodies: early comparison of tacrolimus, mycophenolate mofetil, and steroid dosing, and newer immune-monitoring. Transplantation 2005;80(4):457–65.

[17] McCurry KR, Iacono A, Zeevi A, et al. Early outcomes in human lung transplantation with Thymoglobulin or Campath-1H for recipient pretreatment followed by posttransplant tacrolimus near-monotherapy. J Thorac Cardiovasc Surg 2005;130(2):528–37.

[18] Kaufman DB, Leventhal JR, Gallon LG, et al. Alemtuzumab induction and prednisone-free maintenance immunotherapy in simultaneous pancreas-kidney transplantation comparison with rabbit antithymocyte globulin induction – long-term results. Am J Transplant 2006; 6(2):331–9.

[19] Vathsala A, Ona ET, Tan SY, et al. Randomized trial of alemtuzumab for prevention of graft rejection and preservation of renal function after kidney transplantation. Transplantation 2005;80(6):765–74.

[20] Watson KJE, Gradley JA, Friend PJ, et al. Alemtuzumab (CAMPATH 1H) induction therapy in cadaveric kidney transplantation – efficacy and safety at five years. Am J Transplant 2005;5(6):1347–53.

[21] Campath 1H (Alemtuzumab). Prescribing information. Cambridge (MA): Genzyme Corporation; 2005.

[22] Halloran P. Immunosuppressive drugs for kidney transplantation. N Engl J Med 2004; 351(26):2715–29.

[23] Czock D, Keller F, Rasche FM, et al. Pharmacokinetics and pharmacodynamics of systemically administered glucocorticoids. Clin Pharmacokinet 2005;44(1):61–98.

[24] Holte K, Kehlet H. Perioperative single dose glucocorticoid administration: physiologic effects and clinical implications. J Am Coll Surg 2002;195(5):694–712.

[25] Mittal R, Agarwal SK, Dash SC, et al. Treatment of acute rejection in live related renal allograft recipients: a comparison of three different protocols. Nephron 1997;77(2): 186–9.

[26] Schimmer BP, Parker KL. Adrenocorticotropic hormone; adrenocortical steroids and their synthetic analogs; inhibitors of the synthesis and actions of adrenocortical hormones. In: Brunton LL, editor. Goodman & Gilman's The pharmacologic basis of therapeutics. 11th edition. New York: McGraw-Hill Medical Publishing Division; 2006. p. 1587–612.

[27] Truhan AP, Ahmed RA. Corticosteroids: a review with emphasis on complications of prolonged systemic therapy. Ann Allergy 1989;62:375–90.

[28] Boots JMM, Christiaans MHL, van Hooff JP. Effect of immunosuppressive agents on long-term survival of renal transplant recipients – focus on cardiovascular risk. Drugs 2004; 64(18):2047–73.

[29] Bostom AD, Brown RS, Chavers BM, et al. Prevention of post-transplant cardiovascular disease—report and recommendations of an Ad Hoc Group. Am J Transplant 2002;2: 491–500.

[30] Bromberg JS, Baliga P, Cofer JP, et al. Stress steroids are not required for patients receiving a renal allograft and undergoing operation. J Am Coll Surg 1995;180(5):532–6.

[31] Axelrod L. Perioperative management of patients treated with glucocorticoids. Endocrinol Metab Clin N Am 2003;32:367–83.

[32] Dunn CJ, Wagstaff AJ, Perry CM, et al. Cyclosporin: an updated review of the pharmacokinetic properties, clinical efficacy and tolerability of a microemulsion-based formulation (Neoral) in organ transplantation. Drugs 2001;61(13):1957–2016.

[33] Scott LJ, McKeage K, Keam SJ, et al. Tacrolimus: a further update of its use in the management of organ transplantation. Drugs 2003;63(12):1247–97.

[34] Sandimmune (Cyclosporine). Prescribing information. East Hanover (NJ): Novartis Pharmaceuticals Corporation; 2005.

[35] Prograf (Tacrolimus). Prescribing information. Deerfield (IL): Astella Pharma US, Inc.; 2005.

[36] Margreiter R. Efficacy and safety of tacrolimus compared with ciclosporin microemulsion in renal transplantation: a randomized multicenter study. Lancet 2002;359(9308):741–6.

[37] Ahsan N, Johnson C, Gonwa T, et al. Randomized trial of tacrolimus plus mycophenolate mofetil or azathioprine versus cyclosporine oral solution (modified) plus mycophenolate mofetil after cadaveric kidney transplantation: results at 2 years. Transplantation 2001; 72(2):245–50.

[38] Gonwa T, Johnson C, Ahsan N, et al. Randomized trial of tacrolimus + mycophenolate mofetil or azathioprine versus cyclosporine + mycophenolate mofetil after cadaveric kidney transplantation: results at three years. Transplantation 2003;75(12):2048–53.

[39] Neylan JF. Racial differences in renal transplantation after immunosuppression with tacrolimus versus cyclosporine. Transplantation 1998;65(4):515–23.

[40] McDiarmid S. The necessity for steroid induction or long-term maintenance after liver transplantation: the argument against. Transplant Proc 1998;30(4):1449–51.

[41] Woodle ES, Alloway RR, Buell JF, et al. Multivariate analysis of risk factors for acute rejection in early corticosteroid cessation regimens under modern immunosuppression. Am J Transplant 2005;5(11):2740–4.

[42] Ter Meulen CG, van Riemsdijk I, Hene RJ, et al. Steroid-withdrawal at 3 days after renal transplantation with anti-IL-2 receptor α therapy: a prospective, randomized, multicenter study. Am J Transplant 2004;4(5):803–10.

[43] Rostaing L, Cantarovich D, Mourad G, et al. Corticosteroid-free immunosuppression with tacrolimus, mycophenolate mofetil and daclizumab induction in renal transplantation. Transplantation 2005;79(7):807–14.

[44] Mancinelli LM, Frassetto L, Floren LC, et al. The pharmacokinetics and metabolic disposition of tacrolimus: a comparison across ethnic groups. Clin Pharmacol Ther 2001;69(1): 24–31.

[45] Mancinelli LM, Frassetto L, Floren LC, et al. The pharmacokinetics and metabolic disposition of tacrolimus: a comparison across ethnic groups. Clin Pharmacol Ther 2001;69(1): 24–31.

[46] MacPhee IAM, Fredericks S, Tai T, et al. Tacrolimus pharmacogenetics: polymorphisms associated with expression of cytochrome P4503A5 and p-glycoprotein correlate with dose requirement. Transplantation 2002;74(11):1486–9.

[47] Venkatakrishnan K, von Moltke LL, Greenblatt DJ. Effects of the antifungal agents on oxidative drug metabolism. Clin Pharmacokinet 2000;38(2):111–80.

[48] Lemahieu W, Maes B, Verbeke K, et al. Cytochrome P450 3A4 and p-glycoprotein activity and assimilation of tacrolimus in transplant patients with persistent diarrhea. Am J Transplant 2005;5(6):1383–91.

[49] Chapman JR, O'Connell PJ, Nankivell BJ. Chronic renal allograft dysfunction. J Am Soc Nephrol 2005;16(10):3015–26.

[50] Stratta P, Canavese C, Quaglia M, et al. Posttransplantation chronic renal damage in nonrenal transplant recipients. Kidney Int 2005;68(4):1453–63.

[51] National Institute of Health. National Heart, Lung and Blood Institute. Third Report of the National Cholesterol Education Program (NCEP) Expert Panel on Detection, Evaluation, and Treatment of High Blood Cholesterol in Adults (Adult Treatment Panel III). NIH Publication No. 02–5215, September 2002.

[52] Artz MA, Boots JM, Ligtenberg G, et al. Conversion from cyclosporine to tacrolimus improves quality-of-life indices, renal graft function, and cardiovascular risk profile. Am J Transplant 2004;4(6):937–45.

[53] Backman LA. Post-transplant diabetes mellitus: the last 10 years with tacrolimus. Nephrol Dial Transplant 2004;19(suppl 6):vi13–6.

[54] Imuran (Azathioprine). Prescribing info. San Diego (CA): Prometheus Laboratories, Inc.; 2005.

[55] Murrell GA, Rapeport WG. Clinical pharmacokinetics of allopurinol. Clin Pharmacokinet 1986;11(5):343–53.

[56] Allison AC, Eugui EM. Mechanisms of action of mycophenolate mofetil in preventing acute and chronic allograft rejection. Transplantation 2005;80(2S):S181–90.

[57] Cellcept (Mycophenolate mofetil): complete product information. Nutley (NJ): Roche Laboratories, Inc.; 2004.

[58] Neylan JF. Immunosuppressive therapy in high-risk transplant patients: dose-dependent efficacy of mycophenolate mofetil in African-American renal allograft recipients. US Renal Transpalnt Mycophenolate Mofetil Study Group. Transplantation 1997;64(9): 1277–82.

[59] Bullingham RES, Nicholls AJ, Kamm BR. Clinical pharmacokinetics of mycophenolate mofetil. Clin Pharmacokinet 1998;34(5):429–55.

[60] Meier-Kriesche HU, Shaw LM, Korecka M, et al. Pharmacokinetics of mycophenolic acid in renal insufficiency. Ther Drug Monit 2000;22(1):27–30.

[61] Behrand M. Adverse gastrointestinal effects of mycophenolate mofetil. Drug Saf 2001;24(9): 645–63.

[62] Tricontinental Mycophenolate Mofetil Renal Transplantation Study Group. A blinded, randomized clinical trial of mycophenolate mofetil for the prevention of acute rejection in cadaveric renal transplantation. Transplantation 1996;61(7):1029–37.

[63] Salvadori M, Holzer H, de Mattos A, et al. Enteric-coated mycophenolate sodium is therapeutically equivalent to mycophenolate mofetil in de novo kidney transplant recipients. Am J Transplant 2003;4:231–6.

[64] Curran MP, Keating GM. Mycophenolate sodium delayed released: Prevention of renal transplant rejection. Drugs 2005;65(6):799–805.

[65] Budde K, Curtis J, Knoll G, et al. Enteric-coated mycophenolate sodium can be safely administered in maintenance renal transplant patients: Results of a 1-year study. Am J Transplant 2003;4:237–43.

[66] van Gelder T, Shaw LM. The rationale for and limitations of therapeutic drug monitoring for mycophenolate mofetil in transplantation. Transplantation 2005;80:S244–53.

[67] Borrows R, Chusney G, Loucaidou M, et al. Mycophenolic acid 12-h trough level monitoring in renal transplantation: association with acute rejection and toxicity. Am J Transplant 2006;6:121–8.

[68] Shaw LM, Nawrocki A, Korecka M, et al. Using established immunosuppressant therapy effectively. Ther Drug Monit 2004;26:347–51.

[69] Hubner GI, Eismann R, Sziegoleit W. Drug interaction between mycophenolate mofetil and tacrolimus detectable within therapeutic mycophenolic acid monitoring in renal transplant patients. Ther Drug Monit 1999;21(5):536–9.

[70] Zucker K, Rosen A, Tsaroucha L, et al. Augmentation of mycophenolate mofetil pharmacokinetics in renal transplant patients receiving Prograf and Cellcept in combination therapy. Transplant Proc 1997;29(1–2):334–6.

[71] Van Gelder T, Klupp J, Barten MJ, et al. Comparison of the effects of tacrolimus and cyclosporine on the pharmacokinetics of mycophenolic acid. Ther Drug Monit 2001;23(2):119–28.

[72] Cattaneo D, Merlini S, Zenoni S, et al. Influence of co-medication with sirolimus or cyclosporine on mycophenolic acid pharmacokinetic in kidney transplantation. Am J Transplant 2005;5(12):2937–44.

[73] Zucker K, Tsaroucha A, Olson L, et al. Evidence that tacrolimus augments the bioavailability of mycophenolate mofetil through the inhibitor of mycophenolic acid glucuronidation. Ther Drug Monit 1999;21(1):35–43.

[74] Cattaneo D, Perico N, Gaspari F, et al. Glucocorticoids interfere with mycophenolate mofetil bioavailability in kidney transplantation. Kidney Int 2002;62:1060–7.

[75] Naderer OJ, Dupuis RE, Heinzen EL, et al. The influence of norfloxacin and metronidazole on the disposition of mycophenolate mofetil. J Clin Pharmacol 2005;45(2):219–26.

[76] Watson CJE, Firth J, Williams PF, et al. A randomized controlled trial of late conversion from calcineurin inhibitor-based to sirolimus-based immunosuppression following renal transplantation. Am J Transplant 2005;5:2496–503.

[77] Bumbea V, Kamar N, Ribes D, et al. Long-term results in renal transplant patients with allograft dysfunction after switching from calcineurin inhibitors to sirolimus. Nephrol Dial Transplant 2005;20:2517–23.

[78] Fairbanks KD, Eustace JA, Fine D, et al. Renal function improves in liver transplant recipients when switched from a calcineurin inhibitor to sirolimus. Liver Transpl 2003;9(10):1079–85.

[79] Snell GI, Levvey BJ, Chin W, et al. Sirolimus allows renal recovery in lung and heart transplant recipients with chronic renal impairment. J Heart Lung Transplant 2002;21(5):540–6.

[80] Guba M, Graeb C, Gauch KW, et al. Pro- and anti-cancer effects of immunosuppressive agents used in organ transplantation. Transplantation 2004;77(12):1777–82.

[81] Kauffman HM, Cherikh WS, Cheng Y, et al. Maintenance immunosuppression with target-of-rapamycin inhibitors is associated with a reduced incidence of de novo malignancies. Transplantation 2005;80(7):883–9.

[82] Fung J, Kelly D, Kadry Z, et al. Immunosuppression in liver transplantation. Liver Transpl 2005;11(3):267–80.

[83] Groetzner J, Kur F, Spelsberg F, et al. Airway anastomosis complications in de novo lung transplantation with sirolimus-based immunosuppression. J Heart Lung Transplant 2004;23(5):632–8.

[84] King-Biggs MB, Dunitz JM, Park SJ, et al. Airway anastomotic dehiscence associated with use of sirolimus immediately after lung transplantation. Transplantation 2003;75(9):1437–43.

[85] Fortin MC, Raymond MA, Madore F, et al. Increased risk of thrombotic microangiopathy in patients receiving a cyclosporine-sirolimus combination. Am J Transplant 2004;4(6): 946–52.

[86] Sirolimus (Rapamune). Prescribing information. Philadelphia (PA): Wyeth Pharmaceuticals, Inc.; 2005.

[87] Mahalati K, Kahan BD. Clinical pharmacokinetics of sirolimus. Clin Pharmacokinet 2001; 40(8):573–85.

[88] Kuypers DRJ. Benefit-risk assessment of sirolimus in renal transplantation. Drug Saf 2005; 28(2):153–81.

[89] McTaggert RA, Gottlieb D, Brooks J, et al. Sirolimus prolongs recovery from delayed graft function after cadaveric renal transplantation. Am J Transplant 2003;3:416–23.

[90] Valente JF, Hricik D, Weigel K, et al. Comparison of sirolimus vs. mycophenolate mofetil on surgical complications and wound healing in adult kidney transplantation. Am J Transplant 2003;3:1128–34.

[91] Haydar AA, Denton M, West A, et al. Sirolimus-induced pneumonitis: three cases and a review of the literature. Am J Transplant 2004;4:137–9.

[92] Morelon E, Stern M, Kreis H. Interstitial pneumontitis associated with sirolimus therapy in renal-transplant recipients. N Engl J Med 2000;343(3):225–6.

[93] Singer SJ, Tiernan R, Sullivan EJ. Interstitial pneumonitis associated with sirolimus therapy in renal-transplant recipients. N Engl J Med 2000;343(24):1815–6.

[94] Pham PTT, Pham PCT, Danovitch GM, et al. Siriolimus-associated pulmonary toxicity. Transplantation 2004;77(8):1215–20.

[95] Tedesco-Silva H, Mourad G, Kahan BD, et al. FTY720, a novel immunomodulator: efficacy and safety result from the first phase 2A study in de novo renal transplantation. Transplantation 2004;77(12):1826–33.

[96] Pearson TC, Alexander DZ, Winn KJ, et al. Transplantation tolerance induced by CTLA4-Ig. Transplantation 1994;57(12):1701–6.

[97] Williams JW, Mital D, Chong A, et al. Experiences with leflunomide in solid organ transplantation. Transplantation 2002;73(3):358–66.

[98] Williams JW, Javaid B, Kadambi PB, et al. Leflunomide for polyomavirus type BK nephropathy. N Engl J Med 2005;352(11):1157–8.

[99] Savikko J, Von Willebrand E, Hayry P. Leflunomide analogue FK778 is vasculoprotective independent of its immunosuppressive effect: potential applications for restenosis and chronic rejection. Transplantation 2003;76(3):455–8.

ELSEVIER
SAUNDERS

SURGICAL
CLINICS OF
NORTH AMERICA

Surg Clin N Am 86 (2006) 1185–1194

# Perioperative Concerns for Transplant Recipients Undergoing Nontransplant Surgery

## James Whiting, MD

*Division of Organ Transplantation, Maine Medical Center, 887 Congress Street, Suite 400, Portland, ME 04102, USA*

The likelihood that a nontransplant trained surgeon will encounter a transplant recipient with an unrelated surgical problem is ever increasing. As graft survivals for kidney transplantation have exceeded 90% at 1 year and as long-term graft survival has also improved, the number of patients living with a functioning transplant has doubled over the last 10 years, and as of 2003, there were over 128,000 patients with a functioning kidney transplant [1]. When one considers that the incidence of several common general surgical problems is increased in transplant recipients, it becomes apparent that many of these patients will end up requiring care outside of a transplant center.

In general, surgical problems in the organ transplant recipient can be divided into two categories: problems directly related to the allograft, and those independent of the allograft. Any problem directly related to the allograft should be referred to a transplant center immediately, without exception, and in those situations contact with the transplant center should begin simultaneously with stabilization of the patient. Unfortunately, there are a number of problems where it might not be immediately obvious from the initial clinical presentation that the problem stems directly from the allograft. In addition, even a problem clearly independent of the allograft will require consideration of the patient's immunosuppressed state and careful thought as to how that will effect clinical presentation as well as the response to treatment. At minimum, the physician managing the patient's immunosuppression should be contacted and involved concurrent with any surgical intervention even in what may appear to be the most straightforward of clinical scenarios. Even the subtlest of physical signs and symptoms can be the

---

*E-mail address:* whitij@mmc.org

0039-6109/06/$ - see front matter © 2006 Elsevier Inc. All rights reserved.
doi:10.1016/j.suc.2006.06.011 *surgical.theclinics.com*

harbinger of significant underlying pathophysiology in an immunosuppressed patient. There is no substitute for experience in the care of an ill patient on immunosuppressive therapy.

## Preoperative considerations

In general, preoperative considerations in a transplant recipient are usually independent of the type of transplant and differ little from other patients.

Underlying cardiac status should be carefully assessed before any operation. For a detailed discussion of preoperative cardiac evaluation in the transplant recipient, please refer to the article, "Medical Evaluation and Clearance for Surgery after Transplantation" in this edition. The immunosuppressed state should be considered a cardiac risk factor at least as important as other factors such as hypertension or hyperlipidemia [2]. Beta blockade has been demonstrated as effective in decreasing perioperative cardiac morbidity in general surgical patients [3,4], and should at least be considered in any transplant patient about to undergo a major general surgical procedure.

Preoperative antibiotics have not been extensively studied in transplant recipients undergoing general surgery operations. In general, the recommendations of the National Surgical Infection Project should be followed, and transplant recipients should be considered "at-risk hosts" in this context [5]. This would mean prophylactic antibiotics in virtually all cases, including clean cases. There are no data to suggest a different bacteriology of surgical site infections in transplant patients who sustain postoperative complications, and thus, we recommend using the same antibiotics recommended for the general population and not expanding coverage to unusual or opportunistic organisms. As usual, they should be administered within the first hour before incision [6].

The issue of whether to use stress dose steroid prophylaxis in transplant patients who have chronically been treated with corticosteroids is somewhat controversial. The practice of administering supraphysiologic doses of glucocorticoids perioperatively to patients who have been on steroids chronically, stems from several anecdotal reports of refractory perioperative hypotension and even death in this population, which was attributed to adrenal unresponsiveness [7]. Although it is true that many patients who have been on chronic steroids will exhibit hypothalamic pituitary axis suppression, the actual incidence of a perioperative hypotensive crisis is probably only about 1% [8]. Counterbalancing this, the risks associated with high-dose steroids include wound breakdown, psychiatric disturbances, and detrimental interactions with anesthetic agents. Several authors have demonstrated the safety of maintaining steroid-dependent patients, including transplant patients, on only their chronic doses of glucocorticoids perioperatively [9]. Despite this, the overall level of data available is poor, as highlighted by a recent review on the topic [8], and therefore, most authors still recommend using perioperative steroid augmentation, although 25 to 75 mg of hydrocortisone over 24 to 48 hours is adequate for all but the largest procedures [10].

There are no data to suggest that immunosuppression alters coagulation factors or the risk of deep vein thrombosis (DVT) after surgery. Indeed, there may well be subpopulations of transplant recipients with higher than normal risk for thromboembolic events, as will be discussed later in this article. As such, standard recommendation of the American College of Chest Physicians [11] should be followed.

## Specific surgical situations

### Biliary disease

The optimal management of biliary disease in transplant recipients and patients awaiting transplantation is an area of controversy. Immunosuppressive agents, particularly cyclosporine, are associated with profound changes in serum lipid profiles [12]. There are also experimental data both in people and animals to suggest that cyclosporine is a cholestatic agent, and that the perturbations in bile composition that result from its administration can be responsible for an increased prevalence of biliary stones [13–17]. Clinically, there does appear to be an increased incidence of symptomatic cholelithiasis posttransplant in thoracic as well as kidney and kidney–pancreas transplant recipients [18–21] (the gallbladder is now routinely removed preimplantation in liver allograft recipients as part of the standard allograft preparation procedure). A transplant patient presenting with biliary symptoms should be treated promptly and aggressively. There are no data to suggest varying from suggested algorithms in the management of common biliary emergencies, such as cholecystitis or gallstone pancreatitis, at least in nonliver transplant recipients. Biliary problems in a liver transplant patient, especially strictures, cholangitis, abscesses, and liver bilomas, are certainly the exception to this principle; all such problems should be better referred to a center with experience in liver transplantation. A second area of concern is certain pancreas transplant patients. There are a number of technical modifications of the pancreas transplant procedure, such as mesenteric venous drainage of the allograft and enteric drainage of the pancreatic secretions, which could bring the allograft into the operative field of a routine laparoscopic cholecystectomy. Caution is indicated before considering operative intervention in any pancreas transplant recipient, and preoperative consultation with the original transplanting institution is recommended. There are several reports in thoracic, kidney, and pancreas transplant recipients indicating that laparoscopic cholecystectomy can be completed safely and with reasonable morbidity in this population [18,22,23].

The most controversial issue in this area is the lack of agreement regarding the risk of symptomatic biliary disease in transplant recipients. This is more than just an academic discussion, as this disagreement fuels a larger disagreement upon whether prophylactic cholecystectomy is indicated in patients awaiting transplant with asymptomatic cholelithiasis. A number of programs routinely screen transplant candidates with ultrasound and recommend prophylactic cholecystectomy based on the assumption that any episode of symptomatic biliary disease and especially cholecystitis will impart a higher risk of morbidity and mortality posttransplant. Unfortunately, unlike in the general population where there are a number of good studies and general agreement on the natural history of asymptomatic and symptomatic gallstones [24–26], all of the available data in transplant recipients consist of small, retrospective studies. Within this small collection the results vary widely [22,23,27–30]. Kao and colleagues [18,31] attempted to address this question, first in a review of the subject, which failed to produce a consensus opinion, and more recently using the tools of decision analysis. They concluded that prophylactic cholecystectomy was warranted in patients awaiting thoracic transplantation, but not kidney or kidney pancreas transplantation. Unfortunately, the authors' conclusion was based on the observation of significantly more complications after treatment of symptomatic biliary disease in heart transplant patients compared with kidney transplant patients. The reasons for these large differences in postoperative morbidity and mortality are not intuitively obvious. Importantly, the strength of these recommendations is limited, as the data used as input for the model consisted of retrospective reports of less than 100 patients. The issue of prophylactic cholecystectomy for transplant candidates remains undecided, with advocates citing reports of posttransplant biliary disease leading to allograft loss and death, and others referring to the paucity of data and favorable outcomes of cholecystectomy after transplantation.

## Wound healing and hernia

There can be little argument that immunosuppression inhibits wound healing after surgical therapy [32–35]. There is a voluminous experimental and clinical body of data detailing some of the mechanisms and effects of steroids, calcineurin inhibitors (cyclosporine and tacrolimus), and antiproliferative agents, only a select few that are referenced here [36–41]. Despite these data, a large number of questions remain when the general surgeon is confronted with a transplant recipient with a hernia or wound-healing issue. The relative contribution of individual immunosuppressive agents to wound problems is unclear [42]. Immunosuppressive agents are used almost exclusively in combination therapy, limiting the opportunity for head-to-head comparison. That being said, mycophenolic mofetil (Cellcept) has been shown in one large retrospective series of transplant wound complications to be associated with increased wound problems compared with azathioprine [33]. Although there is substantial experimental evidence that cyclosporine and tacrolimus impair wound healing [36,38,41], until recently, the agents have been considered indispensable in any postoperative transplantation regimen. As a result, little can be deduced about their relative potency in inhibiting wound healing. Steroids have long been recognized as potent inhibitors of wound healing [39]. Interestingly, in a comparison of obese patients to patients on steroids, obesity was demonstrated to be a more potent risk factor for wound complications than steroids [42]. Unfortunately, there is no simple algorithm guiding immunosuppressive management while trying to promote wound healing in a patient with a general surgical problem. Each patient differs in their underlying nutritional status, ability to combat infection, and requirements for immunosuppression. One special situation is the patient on sirolimus.

Sirolimus is an inhibitor of cellular proliferation and cell-signal transduction that has recently become a significant addition to the immunosuppressive armamentarium [43,44]. It impairs fibroblasts and angiogenesis as well as smooth muscle proliferation [45]. Several retrospective studies have demonstrated extraordinarily high rates of wound complications with the drug as have two prospective studies [32,35,44,46,47]. One group reported more favorable rates of wound complications [48,49], but special caution should be given to any general surgeon planning a general surgical operation on a patient taking the agent. Simple uncomplicated wound closures are unlikely to be affected (although we would caution against absorbable sutures), but if a patient on sirolimus presents with a challenging wound situation where healing by secondary intention is anticipated, there should be serious consideration to at least temporary discontinuation of the drug. It also should be recognized that using sirolimus in conjunction with a second antiproliferative agent such as mycophenolate mofetil may produce additive inhibition of fibroblast and smooth muscle proliferation [45,50], and by extension, impair wound healing.

A natural consequence of impaired wound healing is a higher incidence of incisional hernia, and in fact, this does seem to be the case in transplant recipients. The incidence of incisional hernias in liver transplant patients has been reported as high as 17% [34,51], likely from a combination of immunosuppression and the lingering effects of malnutrition and end-stage liver disease. The incidence of incisional hernia in renal transplant patients is lower, from 3% to 4% [33,52]. Although there are no data specifically examining the risk of incisional hernias in transplant patients subsequently undergoing general surgical procedures, it would stand to reason that it would be more common than in the general population.

Because of an immunosuppressed patient's predilection toward infection, it is understandable that an individual surgeon might be hesitant to place prosthetic mesh to repair a hernia in a transplant recipient. In fact, there are several reports confirming the safe placement of prosthetic materials even in already infected wounds in transplant patients [52–54]. Recently, there has also been interest in using new biomeshes for repair of hernias, and there is at least one report of successful use of these materials in transplant recipients [55].

A word of caution is warranted in renal transplant patients. Inguinal hernias on the side of a renal transplant are vanishingly rare. The retroperitoneal location of the allograft serves as an effective barrier to herniation much of the time. An inguinal mass on the side of a renal transplant should be assumed to be related to the allograft until proven otherwise, as lymphoceles and even posttransplant lymphoproliferative disorders can masquerade as inguinal masses in a kidney transplant recipient. Because of the anterior location of the allograft, ultrasonography, accompanied by aspiration or biopsy as indicated, is usually diagnostic.

## Gastrointestinal emergencies

Gastrointestinal complications in the transplant recipient are covered in detail elsewhere in this edition. As such, we will confine our remarks to a few general comments.

Transplant recipients are if anything, more at risk for suffering from gastrointestinal surgical emergencies compared with the general population [56–59]. As with biliary disorders, the clinical presentation may be subtle or completely unexpected due to the masking nature of immunosuppression, and in gener al, one should not hesitate to obtain confirmatory imaging tests in a transplant recipient with any type of gastrointestinal signs and symptoms. Patients need to be treated aggressively, and as with surgical sites, intestinal healing will be impaired [40] and infection rates high. In general, a transplant patient is not a good candidate for nonoperative therapy of a perforated ulcer, complicated diverticulitis, or any other condition that requires a high degree of physiologic wound-healing function.

## Malignancy

The incidences of all cancers, including those of epithelial origin such as adenocarcinoma of the colon, are increased substantially in transplant recipients. A detailed discussion of the interactions between malignancy and immunosuppression are beyond the scope of this article, but there are several excellent reviews [60,61]. In general, one should assume that most tumors in transplant recipients will behave more aggressively, present at a more advanced stage, and respond not as well to standard treatment. Lymphadenopathy in a transplant recipient should be recognized as a particularly serious sign and addressed aggressively. Biopsy to exclude lymphoma should be immediately considered. Unless there is a clear infectious explanation, a waiting period is not appropriate. There are no data to suggest that amelioration or withdrawal of immunosuppression is helpful in treating tumors of epithelial origin as opposed to tumors of lymphatic origin where manipulation of immunosuppression is a central aspect of care.

## Postoperative considerations and complications

### Venous thromboembolism

Venous thromboembolism is a well-described complication of all general surgical procedures. It is a significant cause of morbidity and mortality in the United States today. The incidence, following different transplant procedures, is quite variable, and there is debate as to whether transplant recipients are at any higher risk than comparable patients undergoing similar operations [62]. It appears that the incidence of thromboembolic complications in this population is at least as high as in the general population. A recent report from the United States Data Registry of over 25,000 renal transplant patients has established that renal transplant recipients with diminished renal function (creatinine clearance $< 30$ cc/min) form an especially high-risk subgroup for venous thromboembolic complications [63]. In addition, there are a number of risk factors for thromboembolic events that are more common in the end-stage renal population such as antiphospholipid antibody syndromes. Last, there may be an association of posttransplant cytomegalovirus (CMV) infection with venous thromboembolic events [64].

Diagnostic and treatment algorithms for DVT and pulmonary embolus should not differ from the general population, nor should protocols aimed at prophylaxis. Despite concerns about placing a foreign body above the outflow of renal transplants, renal transplant patients with DVT who fail anticoagulant therapy should have inferior vena caval filters placed [65].

## Summary

The best piece of advice that can be imparted to any general surgeon encountering a transplant recipient as a patient is to proceed with caution and expect the unexpected. Immunosuppression can mask the presenting signs and symptoms of many disease processes as well as postoperative complications. In general, though, the same attention to detail and careful thought processes that produce superior outcomes in any general surgical patient will be of equal or more value in the transplant recipient. Coordinating this care and the management of perioperative immunosuppression in conjunction with the transplant team is recommended.

## References

[1] Annual Report of the USRDS. Percentages and counts of reported ESRD patients: by treatment modality. Bethesda, MD: National Institutes of Health, National Institute of Diabetes and Digestive and Kidney Diseases; 2006.

[2] Kasiske BL, Guijarro C, Massy ZA, et al. Cardiovascular disease after renal transplantation. J Am Soc Nephrol 1996;7:158–65.

[3] Auerbach AD, Goldman L. Beta-blockers and reduction of cardiac events in noncardiac surgery: scientific review. JAMA 2002;287:1435–44.

[4] McGory ML, Maggard MA, Ko CY. A meta-analysis of perioperative beta blockade: what is the actual risk reduction? Surgery 2005;138:171–9.

[5] Bratzler DW, Houck PM. Antimicrobial prophylaxis for surgery: an advisory statement from the National Surgical Infection Prevention Project. Am J Surg 2005;189:395–404.

[6] Bratzler DW, Houck PM, Richards C, et al. Use of antimicrobial prophylaxis for major surgery: baseline results from the National Surgical Infection Prevention Project. Arch Surg 2005;140:174–82.

[7] Kehlet H. A rational approach to dosage and preparation of parenteral glucocorticoid substitution therapy during surgical procedures. A short review. Acta Anaesthesiol Scand 1975; 19:260–4.

[8] Brown CJ, Buie WD. Perioperative stress dose steroids: do they make a difference? J Am Coll Surg 2001;193:678–86.

[9] Bromberg JS, Baliga P, Cofer JB, et al. Stress steroids are not required for patients receiving a renal allograft and undergoing operation. J Am Coll Surg 1995;180:532–6.

[10] Salem M, Tainsh RE Jr, Bromberg J, et al. Perioperative glucocorticoid coverage. A reassessment 42 years after emergence of a problem. Ann Surg 1994;219:416–25.

[11] Geerts WH, Pineo GF, Heit JA, et al. Prevention of venous thromboembolism: the Seventh ACCP Conference on Antithrombotic and Thrombolytic Therapy. Chest 2004;126: 338S–400S.

[12] Hilbrands LB, Demacker PN, Hoitsma AJ, et al. The effects of cyclosporine and prednisone on serum lipid and (apo)lipoprotein levels in renal transplant recipients. J Am Soc Nephrol 1995;5:2073–81.

[13] Cao S, Cox K, So SS, et al. Potential effect of cyclosporin A in formation of cholesterol gallstones in pediatric liver transplant recipients. Dig Dis Sci 1997;42:1409–15.

[14] Moran D, De Buitrago JM, Fernandez E, et al. Inhibition of biliary glutathione secretion by cyclosporine A in the rat: possible mechanisms and role in the cholestasis induced by the drug. J Hepatol 1998;29:68–77.

[15] Hulzebos CV, Bijleveld CM, Stellaard F, et al. Cyclosporine A-induced reduction of bile salt synthesis associated with increased plasma lipids in children after liver transplantation. Liver Transpl 2004;10:872–80.

[16] Sutherland FR, Preshaw RM, Shaffer EA. The effect of cyclosporine and liver autotransplantation on bile flow and composition in dogs. Transplantation 1993;55:237–42.

[17] Chan FK, Shaffer EA. Cholestatic effects of cyclosporine in the rat. Transplantation 1997; 63:1574–8.

[18] Kao LS, Kuhr CS, Flum DR. Should cholecystectomy be performed for asymptomatic cholelithiasis in transplant patients? J Am Coll Surg 2003;197:302–12.

[19] Alberu J, Gatica M, Cachafeiro-Vilar M, et al. Asymptomatic gallstones and duration of cyclosporine use in kidney transplant recipients. Rev Invest Clin 2001;53:396–400.

[20] Spes CH, Angermann CE, Beyer RW, et al. Increased incidence of cholelithiasis in heart transplant recipients receiving cyclosporine therapy. J Heart Transplant 1990;9:404–7.

[21] Weinstein S, Lipsitz EC, Addonizio L, et al. Cholelithiasis in pediatric cardiac transplant patients on cyclosporine. J Pediatr Surg 1995;30:61–4.

[22] Jackson T, Treleaven D, Arlen D, et al. Management of asymptomatic cholelithiasis for patients awaiting renal transplantation. Surg Endosc 2005;19:510–3.

[23] Lord RV, Ho S, Coleman MJ, et al. Cholecystectomy in cardiothoracic organ transplant recipients. Arch Surg 1998;133:73–9.

[24] Gracie WA, Ransohoff DF. The natural history of silent gallstones: the innocent gallstone is not a myth. N Engl J Med 1982;307:798–800.

[25] Ransohoff DF, Gracie WA. Treatment of gallstones. Ann Intern Med 1993;119:606–19.

[26] Friedman GD. Natural history of asymptomatic and symptomatic gallstones. Am J Surg 1993;165:399–404.
[27] Bhatia DS, Bowen JC, Money SR, et al. The incidence, morbidity, and mortality of surgical procedures after orthotopic heart transplantation. Ann Surg 1997;225:686–93.
[28] Graham SM, Flowers JL, Schweitzer E, et al. The utility of prophylactic laparoscopic cholecystectomy in transplant candidates. Am J Surg 1995;169:44–8.
[29] Melvin WS, Meier DJ, Elkhammas EA, et al. Prophylactic cholecystectomy is not indicated following renal transplantation. Am J Surg 1998;175:317–9.
[30] Peterseim DS, Pappas TN, Meyers CH, et al. Management of biliary complications after heart transplantation. J Heart Lung Transplant 1995;14:623–31.
[31] Kao LS, Flowers C, Flum DR. Prophylactic cholecystectomy in transplant patients: a decision analysis. J Gastrointest Surg 2005;9:965–72.
[32] Dean PG, Lund WJ, Larson TS, et al. Wound-healing complications after kidney transplantation: a prospective, randomized comparison of sirolimus and tacrolimus. Transplantation 2004;77:1555–61.
[33] Humar A, Ramcharan T, Denny R, et al. Are wound complications after a kidney transplant more common with modern immunosuppression? Transplantation 2001;72:1920–3.
[34] Gomez R, Hidalgo M, Marques E, et al. Incidence and predisposing factors for incisional hernia in patients with liver transplantation. Hernia 2001;5:172–6.
[35] Troppmann C, Pierce JL, Gandhi MM, et al. Higher surgical wound complication rates with sirolimus immunosuppression after kidney transplantation: a matched-pair pilot study. Transplantation 2003;76:426–9.
[36] Fishel R, Barbul A, Wasserkrug HL, et al. Cyclosporine A impairs wound healing in rats. J Surg Res 1983;34:572–5.
[37] Mohacsi PJ, Tuller D, Hulliger B, et al. Different inhibitory effects of immunosuppressive drugs on human and rat aortic smooth muscle and endothelial cell proliferation stimulated by platelet-derived growth factor or endothelial cell growth factor. J Heart Lung Transplant 1997;16:484–92.
[38] Petri JB, Schurk S, Gebauer S, et al. Cyclosporine A delays wound healing and apoptosis and suppresses activin beta-A expression in rats. Eur J Dermatol 1998;8:104–13.
[39] Anstead GM. Steroids, retinoids, and wound healing. Adv Wound Care 1998;11:277–85.
[40] Zeeh J, Inglin R, Baumann G, et al. Mycophenolate mofetil impairs healing of left-sided colon anastomoses. Transplantation 2001;71:1429–35.
[41] Schaffer M, Fuchs N, Volker J, et al. Differential effect of tacrolimus on dermal and intestinal wound healing. J Invest Surg 2005;18:71–9.
[42] Sugerman HJ, Kellum JM Jr, Reines HD, et al. Greater risk of incisional hernia with morbidly obese than steroid-dependent patients and low recurrence with prefascial polypropylene mesh. Am J Surg 1996;171:80–4.
[43] Sehgal SN. Rapamune (RAPA, rapamycin, sirolimus): mechanism of action immunosuppressive effect results from blockade of signal transduction and inhibition of cell cycle progression. Clin Biochem 1998;31:335–40.
[44] Kahan BD. Efficacy of sirolimus compared with azathioprine for reduction of acute renal allograft rejection: a randomised multicentre study. The Rapamune US Study Group. Lancet 2000;356:194–202.
[45] Gregory CR, Huang X, Pratt RE, et al. Treatment with rapamycin and mycophenolic acid reduces arterial intimal thickening produced by mechanical injury and allows endothelial replacement. Transplantation 1995;59:655–61.
[46] Valente JF, Hricik D, Weigel K, et al. Comparison of sirolimus vs. mycophenolate mofetil on surgical complications and wound healing in adult kidney transplantation. Am J Transplant 2003;3:1128–34.
[47] Langer RM, Kahan BD. Incidence, therapy, and consequences of lymphocele after sirolimus–cyclosporine–prednisone immunosuppression in renal transplant recipients. Transplantation 2002;74:804–8.

[48] Flechner SM, Goldfarb D, Modlin C, et al. Kidney transplantation without calcineurin inhibitor drugs: a prospective, randomized trial of sirolimus versus cyclosporine. Transplantation 2002;74:1070–6.

[49] Flechner SM, Zhou L, Derweesh I, et al. The impact of sirolimus, mycophenolate mofetil, cyclosporine, azathioprine, and steroids on wound healing in 513 kidney-transplant recipients. Transplantation 2003;76:1729–34.

[50] Jolicoeur EM, Qi S, Xu D, et al. Combination therapy of mycophenolate mofetil and rapamycin in prevention of chronic renal allograft rejection in the rat. Transplantation 2003;75:54–9.

[51] Janssen H, Lange R, Erhard J, et al. Causative factors, surgical treatment and outcome of incisional hernia after liver transplantation. Br J Surg 2002;89:1049–54.

[52] Mazzucchi E, Nahas WC, Antonopoulos I, et al. Incisional hernia and its repair with polypropylene mesh in renal transplant recipients. J Urol 2001;166:816–9.

[53] Muller V, Lehner M, Klein P, et al. Incisional hernia repair after orthotopic liver transplantation: a technique employing an inlay/onlay polypropylene mesh. Langenbecks Arch Surg 2003;388:167–73.

[54] Antonopoulos IM, Nahas WC, Mazzucchi E, et al. Is polypropylene mesh safe and effective for repairing infected incisional hernia in renal transplant recipients? Urology 2005;66:874–7.

[55] Catena F, Ansaloni L, Leone A, et al. Lichtenstein repair of inguinal hernia with Surgisis inguinal hernia matrix soft-tissue graft in immunodepressed patients. Hernia 2005;9:29–31.

[56] Steed DL, Brown B, Reilly JJ, et al. General surgical complications in heart and heart–lung transplantation. Surgery 1985;98:739–45.

[57] Bardaxoglou E, Maddern G, Ruso L, et al. Gastrointestinal surgical emergencies following kidney transplantation. Transpl Int 1993;6:148–52.

[58] Smith PC, Slaughter MS, Petty MG, et al. Abdominal complications after lung transplantation. J Heart Lung Transplant 1995;14:44–51.

[59] Maurer JR. The spectrum of colonic complications in a lung transplant population. Ann Transplant 2000;5:54–7.

[60] Whiting JF, Hanto DW. Cancer in recipients of organ allografts. In: Racusen LC, Solez K, Burdick JF, editors. Kidney transplant rejection. New York: Marcel Dekker; 1998. p. 577–604.

[61] Buell JF, Gross TG, Woodle ES. Malignancy after transplantation. Transplantation 2005;80:S254–64.

[62] Humar A, Johnson EM, Gillingham KJ, et al. Venous thromboembolic complications after kidney and kidney–pancreas transplantation: a multivariate analysis. Transplantation 1998;65:229–34.

[63] Abbott KC, Cruess DF, Agodoa LY, et al. Early renal insufficiency and late venous thromboembolism after renal transplantation in the United States. Am J Kidney Dis 2004;43:120–30.

[64] Kazory A, Ducloux D, Coaquette A, et al. Cytomegalovirus-associated venous thromboembolism in renal transplant recipients: a report of 7 cases. Transplantation 2004;77:597–9.

[65] Jarrell BE, Szentpetery S, Mendez-Picon G, et al. Greenfield filter in renal transplant patients. Arch Surg 1981;116:930–2.

ELSEVIER
SAUNDERS

SURGICAL
CLINICS OF
NORTH AMERICA

Surg Clin N Am 86 (2006) 1195–1206

# Gastrointestinal Complications Following Transplantation

## Amitabh Gautam, MD

*Brown Medical School, Division of Organ Transplantation, Rhode Island Hospital,*
*593 Eddy Street, Providence, RI 02903, USA*

Organ transplantation has emerged as the preferred treatment modality for end-stage liver, kidney, heart, and lung diseases. Approximately 27,000 organs are transplanted every year in the United States, establishing a large cohort of patients with a wide variety of medical conditions who require chronic immunosuppression. Because gastrointestinal complaints occur in 30% to 40% of these patients and serious gastrointestinal conditions occur in 10% of these patients, most general surgeons will encounter transplant recipients presenting with gastrointestinal symptoms. This review will focus on some unique features of gastrointestinal complications occurring in this population.

The gastrointestinal tract accounts for a large component of non–allograft-related complications seen after all types of solid organ transplantation [1–4] and is responsible for considerable morbidity and mortality associated with transplantation. Gastrointestinal diseases such as peptic ulcers, colonic diverticulosis, or cholelithiasis can be present before organ transplantation. These conditions can be exacerbated by immunosuppression or result in increased morbidity and mortality when pathologic conditions develop in an immunosuppressed host. Immunosuppressive and other drugs required after transplantation often have gastrointestinal side effects or they can modify the symptoms and presentation of gastrointestinal diseases in these patients. Non-specific immunosuppression also predisposes patients to infection by a variety of gastrointestinal viral, bacterial, fungal, and parasitic pathogens and could increase the severity of disease from common pathogens.

*E-mail address:* amitabh_gautam@brown.edu

0039-6109/06/$ - see front matter © 2006 Elsevier Inc. All rights reserved.
doi:10.1016/j.suc.2006.06.006      *surgical.theclinics.com*

## Oral lesions

Cyclosporine-induced gingival hyperplasia is common and is perhaps caused by drug-induced decreased collagenolytic activity in the gum [5]. Treatment consists of improving oral hygiene [6], and oral azithromycin can be helpful in some cases [7]. Tacrolimus or sirolimus, which do not cause gingival hyperplasia, can be substituted for cyclosporine. Oral ulcers arise in transplant recipients typically as a consequence of viral infections such as cytomegalovirus (CMV) and herpes simplex virus (HSV). Therapy consists of antiviral therapy often accompanied by reduction in immunosuppression. Aphthous stomatitis is particularly common in patients receiving sirolimus and might require discontinuation of this medication [8]. The use of immunosuppressive agents predisposes patients to oral candidiasis either alone or in association with esophageal infection. Prophylaxis with nystatin or clotrimazole troches is recommended, but breakthrough or resistant infections arise occasionally.

Epstein-Barr virus (EBV)-associated oral hairy leucoplakia, identified as a grayish-white lesion on the lateral border of the tongue that cannot be scraped off, might display vertical ridges and does not respond to antimycotic treatment [6]. Lesions of Kaposi's sarcoma, mucosal warts, and a number of other malignant and premalignant conditions have been reported in transplant patients [9]. A biopsy is indicated for nonhealing lesions and any lesion that is suspicious for malignancy.

## Peptic ulcer disease

Historically, peptic ulcer disease after transplantation carried a grim prognosis. The mortality from gastroduodenal ulcers in renal transplant recipients was greater more than 40% before the use of H2 antagonists and proton pump inhibitors [10]. The higher incidence of peptic ulcers in kidney transplant recipients might be related to a higher incidence of peptic lesions and *Helicobacter pylori* infection in patients who have chronic renal failure [11]. In the current era there has been a decrease in both the incidence and severity of peptic ulcer disease in transplant recipients, which reflects the changing epidemiology of peptic ulcer disease in the general population, aggressive screening of transplant candidates, and active treatment of pre-existing disease with H2 receptor antagonists or proton pump inhibitors. After transplantation, most protocols include prophylaxis with these drugs for a variable period of time [12]. There appears to be no clear benefit of one class of antacid drug over another for gastrointestinal prophylaxis [13]. There is also controversy for how long this treatment is necessary after transplantation.

Increasingly, *H pylori* is recognized as the key to the pathogenesis of peptic ulcer disease. Forty adult recipients for living donor liver transplantation were screened for absence of pre-existing peptic ulcer disease by history and upper gastrointestinal endoscopy [14]. Twenty-five (62.5%) recipients tested positive for *H pylori* and six recipients developed duodenal ulcers after transplantation. None of the *H pylori*-negative recipients developed peptic ulcers, suggesting that preoperative screening and prompt treatment might eliminate post-transplant disease. Candidates for transplantation who have prior history or symptoms suggestive of peptic ulcer should have an upper gastrointestinal endoscopy for evaluation of the lesion and ensuring that the lesion has healed completely before transplantation [15].

The relationship of corticosteroids to peptic ulcer disease is unclear. Some authors have implicated immunosuppressive medications, especially steroids, in the genesis of peptic ulcers. The majority of acute rejection episodes in the transplanted organ are treated by brief pulses of high-dose steroids, which further increase the risk of development of peptic ulcers [16,17]. It is recommended that patients resume or increase anti-ulcer prophylaxis during this period; however, a meta-analysis of patients on corticosteroids showed that peptic ulcer was a rare complication of steroid therapy [18]. Indeed, the infectious etiology of most peptic disease suggests that immunosuppression, and not corticosteroids per se, might exacerbate ulcer disease. To the benefit of transplant recipients, the simultaneous development of more specific immunosuppression and effective prophylaxis for peptic ulcer disease has obscured this association. Currently it appears that a history of gastritis or peptic disease is not a contraindication to steroid therapy. Symptomatic peptic disease can increase with the administration of immunosuppressive medications, and evaluation for *H pylori* infection and endoscopy should be undertaken. As in the general population, most cases are treatable by antacids and antibiotic therapy as indicated.

## Biliary tract disease

Pancreaticobiliary disease is highly prevalent in heart transplant recipients, and emergent surgery for acute biliary tree complications can have a mortality of up to 29% [19,20]. Given the high complication rate for symptomatic biliary disease after heart transplantation, most centers advocate screening candidates before listing; however, cholecystectomy in patients who have advanced heart failure can also be problematic. A retrospective series of cardiac transplant candidates proposed that prophylactic cholecystectomy resulted in decreased mortality and significant cost savings compared with treatment of biliary colic, acute cholecystitis, or biliary pancreatitis after transplantation [21].

A strategy of prophylactic cholecystectomy has been studied in patients awaiting renal transplantation. In the absence of large, randomized trials, controversy persists regarding the need for pre-transplant screening for cholelithiasis and performing a cholecystectomy if asymptomatic gallstones are found [22,23]. Pre-transplant screening with ultrasound is effective and non-invasive. Patients who have asymptomatic gallstones found during the evaluation for transplantation can be operated upon with an acceptably low morbidity. There is a perceived increased risk of surgery in patients on chronic immunosuppression; however, a number of small series demonstrate that there is no increased risk of morbidity from cholecystectomy after transplantation [22,24]. The small numbers of patients in these series prohibit firm conclusions but suggest a case-by-case approach in asymptomatic disease and early intervention for symptomatic disease [25].

## Gastrointestinal malignancy

It is generally accepted that the incidence of common gastrointestinal cancers is not increased after transplantation compared with the general population [26]; however, with continued improvement in transplantation outcomes and improved life expectancy, post-transplant malignancy has become an important cause of mortality. A retrospective study of 73,076 kidney and heart transplant recipients to determine the incidence of gastric, colonic, and rectal cancers found that, compared with the general population, there was no increase in the incidence of gastric cancer, a small increase in the incidence of colonic cancer, and a significant reduction in the incidence of rectal cancer [27]. Registry data in the United States similarly suggest little effect of immunosuppression on common gastrointestinal malignancies. Unfortunately, reporting bias, incomplete data, and screening bias in a population that is subject to increased medical follow-up and surveillance complicates the interpretation of registry data. Impaired immunosurveillance of neoplastic cells and depressed antiviral activity are believed to contribute to the added risk of cancer after transplantation [28]. Although it is unclear whether or not the incidence of the most common cancers (lung, breast, colon, prostate) is increased after transplantation, cancers that have a viral pathogenesis are clearly increased in this population. In the gastrointestinal tract this includes a higher incidence of oral and anal malignancies. A Swedish population-based cancer registry study showed a sixfold increase in cancer of the oral cavity in organ transplant recipients [29]. The risk of anal cancer in transplant recipients is markedly raised from 10 to 20 times compared with the general population [29,30]. This is because of increased proliferation of human papilloma virus (HPV) with immunosuppression, which has been implicated as a causal agent for this cancer [26,30].

Post-transplant lymphoproliferative disorder (PTLD) is one of the most common malignancies after transplantation, and the gastrointestinal tract, with its large amount of lymphoid tissue, is affected in many cases [31]. Unlike nodal PTLD, gastrointestinal PTLD can have minimal symptoms in the early phase, and the majority of patients present with the complication of obstruction, bleeding, or perforation [32]. A high index of clinical suspicion is needed and an open or endoscopic biopsy is needed for full histopathologic characterization [33]. Of particular importance in planning therapy are the following characteristics of the lymphoma: monoclonal versus polyclonal, B cell versus T cell, the presence of EBV, and CD20 lymphocytes. Approximately 85% of post-transplant lymphomas are derived from B lymphocytes and most are associated with proliferation of EBV [34]. Transplant recipients without prior exposure to EBV (serologically naïve), particularly children, are at increased risk. Early detection strategies, such as serial measurements of EBV DNA load in peripheral blood samples, are indicated in this population. A rise in the titer should prompt reduction in immunosuppression and heightened surveillance. There might be a role for antiviral treatment in the management of EBV-associated lymphoproliferation. Treatment strategies are based on the severity of disease and the need for immunosuppression to preserve transplant organ function. Therapy typically consists of reducing or ceasing immunosuppression and chemotherapy. Surgery might be required for debulking or to manage complications. Many patients have CD20-positive lymphocytes present and a specific anti-CD20 monoclonal antibody (rituximab) is commonly administered as part of the treatment [35]. The prognosis is variable; however, complete remission is often reported in more than 50% of cases.

## Colonic perforation

The incidence of colonic perforation after transplantation is 1% to 2% and the mortality from this abdominal catastrophe in an immunosuppressed patient is very high (20–38%) [2,36]. Diverticulitis is the most common cause for these perforations, followed by ischemic colitis and CMV colitis, which can co-exist [36–38]. Non-obstructing colonic dilatation can arise in the early postoperative period and can result in right-side colonic perforation [39]. Alterations in the integrity of the colon wall caused by lymphodepletion, retraction on the colon during surgery, and postoperative ileus have been postulated as contributing factors to this complication. Colonoscopy might be helpful in decompressing the colon and preventing a perforation.

The potassium binding resin, sodium polystyrene sulfonate (Kayexalate), used for the treatment of hyperkalemia has been implicated as a cause of ileocolonic or colonic necrosis and perforation [40,41]. The usual clinical scenario involves a patient who has delayed graft function and hyperkalemia following kidney transplantation. Ischemia and necrosis of the colon occur after a Kayexalate–sorbitol enema. Many centers consider the use of Kayexalate in this setting taboo; however, others commonly employ this form of therapy. The few case reports in the literature hardly establish causation.

The role of pre-transplant screening for colonic diverticular disease and prophylactic colectomy has not been established [42]. Treatment of asymptomatic diverticulosis is geared to the prevention of constipation. Referral to a dietician with recommendations for addition of vegetables, fruits, and cereals (bran) to the diet seems prudent. When dietary manipulations are not well tolerated, hydrophilic bulk laxatives are a useful alternative. There is evidence that patients who have polycystic kidney disease have a higher incidence of diverticulosis and a higher incidence of gastrointestinal complications after kidney transplantation [43]. Early surgical intervention is indicated after colonic perforation.

**Gastrointestinal infections**

Because of their non-specific immunosuppression, transplant recipients are susceptible to a number of pathogens—viral, fungal, protozoan, and bacterial, that primarily affect the gastrointestinal tract. The risk of infection itself is determined by the patient's net state of immunosuppression and the presence of anatomic or technical abnormalities and the patient's epidemiological exposures. The causes of infectious disease syndromes vary with the time course from transplantation defined as the perioperative period, early after (months 1–6), and late after transplantation [32]. Perioperative gastrointestinal infections can result from a pre-existing infection in the recipient, donor-transmitted infections, leaks from enteric anastomosis, or from the surgical wound. It is often difficult to distinguish between infection-related and immunosuppression-related gastrointestinal effects during this period. During the first 6 months after transplantation, viral and other opportunistic infections prevail. Beyond 6 months after transplantation, patients who have a good result from the transplant are at risk primarily for community-acquired microbes, including such enteric pathogens as Salmonella. Of the remaining patients, those who have marginal allograft function, repeated hospitalizations, and especially those who have received additional immunosuppression for the treatment of acute rejection remain at greatest risk for opportunistic infection. The infection timeline is helpful in determining whether a gastrointestinal complication is likely to be related to over-immunosuppression, sporadic infection, or a specific effect of an immunosuppressant drug. Fever, inflammatory cells in the stool, abnormalities on endoscopy or computed tomography, and leukocytosis can be useful in the diagnosis but are inconsistent markers for an infectious cause [32].

**Viral infections**

CMV, HSV, adenovirus, and human calicivirus can cause gastrointestinal disease in the transplant recipient. CMV infection is the most common viral infection causing clinical symptoms after transplantation. CMV, like other herpesviruses, produces life-long latent infection. In the immunocompetent host, primary infection is generally asymptomatic. The majority of adults are seropositive for CMV IgG, indicating resolved infection. After transplantation, CMV infection could arise from infected passenger leukocytes within the allograft transplanted into a CMV-naïve recipient (Donor +, Recipient −: D+/R−) or cause superinfection in a CMV-positive recipient (D+/R+) [44]. Latent CMV in a seropositive recipient could also be reactivated and upregulated by immunosuppressive medications. Different types of organ transplantation carry different risks for activation of post-transplantation CMV. The intestines, pancreas, and lungs are associated with the highest risk, followed by liver and heart transplantation, with kidney transplantation causing the least risk [45]. This hierarchy is related to the amount of immunosuppression initially required and the amount of CMV load in the lymphoid and endothelial cells of the transplanted organ. At any time, if additional immunosuppression is required to reverse rejection of the allograft (especially the use of antilymphocyte antibodies) the risk of reactivation of CMV increases dramatically. CMV infection is usually systemic, presenting with viremia and constitutional symptoms such as fatigue, fever, malaise, anorexia, arthralgia, and, classically, leukopenia. In addition, the infection can be localized predominantly to an organ, including any part of the gastrointestinal tract. The gastrointestinal tract is involved in 10% to 30% of patients who have CMV disease [46]. The presentation is usually localized. Patients can present with CMV esophagitis, gastritis, duodenitis, small bowel enteritis, or colitis. Viral infection can produce bleeding, ulceration, diffuse mucosal irritation, and (less commonly) perforation. The symptoms depend on the affected part and can range from dysphagia, nausea, vomiting, abdominal pain, gastrointestinal bleeding, and diarrhea.

The availability of ganciclovir as an effective agent against CMV has led to its widespread use immediately after transplantation and for about 3 months for prophylactic purposes. Valganciclovir, which is a pro-drug of ganciclovir, has much better oral bioavailability and is increasingly being used for both prophylaxis and treatment. A double-blind study of valganciclovir and ganciclovir showed that valganciclovir was as effective as ganciclovir for prevention of CMV disease in high-risk (D+/R−) recipients [47]. Patients receiving valganciclovir also had lower incidence of CMV viremia, and if there was a breakthrough reactivation, they had lower peak CMV loads. CMV prophylaxis should be restarted any time that acute rejection of the allograft is being treated, especially if antilymphocyte preparations are being used. The widespread routine use of post-transplant prophylaxis is changing the epidemiology of the disease, and more cases are seen after CMV prophylaxis has been stopped rather than in the traditional period of the first 6 months after transplantation. Because the clinical features are non-specific, the diagnosis of CMV should be confirmed by laboratory methods. The most sensitive method for detection of CMV in blood, body fluid, or tissue specimen is by amplifying CMV DNA by the polymerase chain reaction. Endoscopy for gastrointestinal symptoms with tissue biopsy is needed for early diagnosis and initiating antiviral treatment. Though rare, late cases of CMV infection, occurring sometimes many years after stable allograft function, have been described [48].

HSV presents with reactivation of the latent virus during periods of intense immunosuppression, typically in the first month after transplantation, as mucocutaneous ulcers involving the oral cavity and pharynx. The esophagus can also be involved, especially during treatment of acute rejection by pulse steroids or antilymphocyte preparations [49]. Symptoms of odynophagia or dysphagia should prompt endoscopy and biopsy for confirmation. Extensive oral infection can be treated by oral acyclovir, but disseminated and severe infections require intravenous therapy.

Other vial pathogens that affect the gastrointestinal tract after transplantation include adenovirus and calicivirus. Both usually cause a mild disease including diarrhea in immunocompetent hosts, but can cause severe disease in immunosuppressed hosts. Calicivirus has also been reported to cause severe enteritis after small bowel transplantation. In those cases a further distinction is often required between viral infection and allograft rejection.

## Fungal infections

The most common fungal gastrointestinal infection in transplant recipients is candidiasis, commonly affecting the oral cavity and the esophagus. The usual presentation is within the first 6 months after transplantation, or later when high-dose steroids are used to treat acute allograft rejection or with the use of broad-spectrum antibiotics. Although *Candida albicans* remains the commonest species, the rate of infection with *Candida glabrata*, *Candida tropicalis*, and *Candida parapsilosis* is increasing, and many of these organisms have antifungal resistance [50]. Presentation is with dysphagia, heartburn, or gastrointestinal bleeding. Endoscopy might show superficial erosions, ulcers, and white nodules or plaques. Diagnosis is made by fungal cultures and histopathologic examination. Treatment is usually by topical nystatin. Intravenous amphotericin might be required for severe infections and if there is fungemia. Because of resistant strains and an improved side effect profile, modern therapy for severe fungal infections has shifted away from amphotericin with more use of caspofungin, posaconazole, and voriconazole. Rarely, upper gastrointestinal infection can progress to severe local tissue destruction, causing esophageal perforation.

## Parasitic infections

Immunosuppressed transplant recipients are susceptible to protozoal infection with *Microsporidium*, *Cryptosporidium*, *Isospora belli*, *Cyclospora*, and *Giardia lamblia*. These infections present with diarrhea, and diagnosis is made with identification of the specific ova on stool examination. Patients might have a long history of chronic episodic diarrhea. The ova of *Cryptosporidium* are very small and require special techniques for its detection. Microscopic examination of biopsy specimen from the intestinal mucosa can show *Cryptosporidium* [51]. In addition to specific chemotherapy, reduction of immunosuppression might be needed for elimination of the parasite.

The nematode *Strongyloides stercoralis* might remain quiescent for several years and present only after the initiation of immunosuppression after transplantation. Interestingly, cyclosporine has anti-helminthic properties and might suppress the parasite. One case report described that hyperinfection with *Strongyloides* occurred after stopping cyclosporine [52].

## Bacterial infections

Bacterial infections of the gastrointestinal tract causing diarrhea are not uncommon in transplant recipients. The causal organisms are *Clostridia difficile*, *Yersinia enterocolitica*, *Campylobacter jejuni*, *Salmonella* sp, and *Listeria monocytogenes* [32]. Up to 50% of transplant patients receiving a therapeutic course of antibiotics develop *C difficile*-associated diarrhea [53]. The disease spectrum is very wide, from diarrhea to febrile enterocolitis and toxic megacolon. Not uncommonly, patients might present with recurrent disease [54]. *C difficile* colitis should be entertained in transplant patients who have a history of diarrhea after antibiotic use and should be treated aggressively before the infection becomes complicated.

## Diarrhea

Diarrhea is a common gastrointestinal complication after transplantation. The etiology could be infection, the direct effect of medications including immunosuppressant drugs and antibiotics, and the surgical procedure itself. A large number of gastrointestinal infections of the gastrointestinal tract can present with diarrhea as a major symptom. An extensive work-up including stool examination and serological studies is needed to diagnose the causative agent. Although diarrhea has been reported with all immunosuppressant medications, mycophenolate mofetil (MMF) is most often associated with frequent gastrointestinal side effects [55]. Up to 27% of patients taking MMF develop gastrointestinal complications, often resulting in discontinuation of the drug. Discontinuation of MMF is not without risk and has been associated with an increased risk of acute rejection and graft loss [56]. Consideration should be given to substituting an alternative agent rather than discontinuing MMF. A multidisciplinary approach is recommended for the management of transplant patients who have gastrointestinal complaints to maintain adequate immunosuppression and preserve allograft integrity while addressing gastrointestinal symptoms. Unlike bone marrow transplantation, graft versus host disease causing diarrhea is a rare complication of solid organ transplantation, being almost exclusively limited to the graft-derived lymphocytes of the small bowel allograft causing intestinal immunologic injury and diarrhea.

## Strategies for management

The etiology of most gastrointestinal complications is complex and involves drug side effects, infective agents, and pre-existing conditions. Early diagnosis and prompt surgical intervention (when necessary) are indicated. Secondary infection and sepsis in immunosuppressed patients can progress rapidly and is commonly fatal. Corticosteroid medications can mask signs and symptoms of serious gastrointestinal pathology, thus a high index of suspicion is needed. Because treatment might involve an alteration in immunosuppression, the transplant team should be contacted and involved as soon as possible. A transplant infectious disease specialist as part of this team is invaluable in coordinating the complex diagnostic and therapeutic maneuvers required in managing these patients. Gastrointestinal endoscopic evaluation should be initiated early, even for relatively minor symptoms. Appropriate tissue specimens might need to be processed for evaluation of an infective component. Early diagnosis, appropriate adjustments in immunosuppressive medications, and prompt therapy reduce morbidity and can be life-saving.

## References

[1] Hoekstra HJ, Hawkins K, de Boer WJ, et al. Gastrointestinal complications in lung transplant survivors that require surgical intervention. Br J Surg 2001;88:433–8.
[2] Sarkio S, Halme L, Kyllonen L, et al. Severe gastrointestinal complications after 1,515 adult kidney transplantations. Transplant Int 2004;17:505–10.
[3] Luckraz H, Goddard M, Charman SC, et al. Early mortality after cardiac transplantation: should we do better? J Heart Lung Transplant 2005;24:401–5.
[4] Goldberg HJ, Hertz MI, Ricciardi R, et al. Colon and rectal complications after heart and lung transplantation. J Am Coll Surg 2006;202:55–61.
[5] Hyland PL, Traynor PS, Myrillas TT, et al. The effects of cyclosporin on the collagenolytic activity of gingival fibroblasts. J Periodontol 2003;74:437–45.
[6] de la Rosa-Garcia E, Mondragon-Padilla A, Irigoyen-Camacho ME, et al. Oral lesions in a group of kidney transplant patients. Med Oral Patol Oral Cir Bucal 2005;10:196–204.
[7] Nash MM, Zaltzman JS. Efficacy of azithromycin in the treatment of cyclosporine-induced gingival hyperplasia in renal transplant recipients. Transplantation 1998;65:1611–5.
[8] van Gelder T, ter Meulen CG, Hene R, et al. Oral ulcers in kidney transplant recipients treated with sirolimus and mycophenolate mofetil. Transplantation 2003;75:788–91.
[9] Seymour RA, Thomason JM, Nolan A. Oral lesions in organ transplant patients. J Oral Pathol Med 1997;26:297–304.
[10] Owens ML, Passaro E, Wilson SE, et al. Treatment of peptic ulcer disease in the renal transplant patient. Ann Surg 1977;186:17–21.
[11] Nardone G, Rocco A, Fiorillo M, et al. Gastroduodenal lesions and *Helicobacter pylori* infection in dyspeptic patients with and without chronic renal failure. Helicobacter 2005;10:53–8.
[12] Helderman JH. Prophylaxis and treatment of gastrointestinal complications following transplantation. Clin Transplant 2001;15(S):29–35.
[13] Skala I, Mareckova O, Vitko S, et al. Prophylaxis of acute gastro duodenal bleeding after renal transplantation. Transplant Int 1997;10:375–8.
[14] Hosotani Y, Kawanami C, Hasegawa K, et al. A role of *Helicobacter pylori* infection in the development of duodenal ulcer after adult living-related liver transplantation. Transplantation 2003;76:702–4.

[15] Kasiske BL, Cangro CB, Hariharan S, et al. The evaluation of renal transplantation candidates: clinical practice guidelines. Am J Transplant 2001;2(S):3–95.

[16] Steger AC, Timoney AS, Griffen S, et al. The influence of immunosuppression on peptic ulceration following renal transplantation and the role of endoscopy. Nephrol Dial Transplant 1990;5:289–92.

[17] Chen KJ, Chen CH, Cheng CH, et al. Risk factors for peptic ulcer disease in renal transplant patients—11 years of experience from a single center. Clin Nephrol 2004;62:14–20.

[18] Conn HO, Poynard T. Corticosteroids and peptic ulcer: meta-analysis of adverse events during steroid therapy. J Intern Med 1994;236:619–32.

[19] Vega KJ, Pina I, Krevsky B. Heart transplantation is associated with an increased risk for pancreaticobiliary disease. Ann Intern Med 1996;124:980–3.

[20] Gupta D, Sakorafas GH, McGregor CG, et al. Management of biliary tract disease in heart and lung transplant patients. Surgery 2000;128:641–9.

[21] Richardson WS, Surowiec WJ, Carter KM, et al. Gallstone disease in heart transplant recipients. Ann Surg 2003;237:273–6.

[22] Melvin WS, Meier DJ, Elkhammas EA, et al. Prophylactic cholecystectomy is not indicated following renal transplantation. Am J Surg 1998;175:317–9.

[23] Graham SM, Flowers JL, Schweitzer E, et al. The utility of prophylactic laparoscopic cholecystectomy in transplant candidates. Am J Surg 1995;169:44–9.

[24] Jackson T, Treleaven D, Arlen D, et al. Management of asymptomatic cholelithiasis for patients awaiting renal transplantation. Surg Endosc 2005;19:510–3.

[25] Kao LS, Flowers C, Flum DR. Prophylactic cholecystectomy in transplant patients: a decision analysis. J Gastrointest Surg 2005;9:965–72.

[26] Penn I. Posttransplant malignancies. Transplant Proc 1999;31:1260–2.

[27] Stewart T, Henderson R, Grayson H, et al. Reduced incidence of rectal cancer, compared to gastric and colonic cancer, in a population of 73,076 men and women chronically immunosuppressed. Clin Cancer Res 1997;3:51–5.

[28] Buell JF, Gross TG, Woodle ES. Malignancy after transplantation. Transplantation 2005; 80(S):S254–64.

[29] Adami J, Gabel H, Lindelof B, et al. Cancer risk following organ transplantation: a nationwide cohort study in Sweden. Br J Cancer 2003;89:1221–7.

[30] Sillman FH, Sentovich S, Shaffer D. Ano-genital neoplasia in renal transplant patients. Ann Transplant 1997;2:59–66.

[31] Swinnen LJ. Diagnosis and treatment of transplant-related lymphoma. Ann Oncol 2000; 11(S):45–8.

[32] Rubin RH. Gastrointestinal infectious disease complications following transplantation and their differentiation from immunosuppressant-induced gastrointestinal toxicities. Clin Transplant 2001;15(S)4:11–22.

[33] Green M. Management of Epstein-Barr virus-induced post-transplant lymphoproliferative disease in recipients of solid organ transplantation. Am J Transplant 2001;1:103–8.

[34] Savage P, Waxman J. Post-transplantation lymphoproliferative disease. QJM 1997;90: 497–503.

[35] Oertel SH, Verschuuren E, Reinke P, et al. Effect of anti-CD 20 antibody rituximab in patients with post-transplant lymphoproliferative disorder (PTLD). Am J Transplant 2005; 5:2901–6.

[36] Stelzner M, Vlahakos DV, Milford EL, et al. Colonic perforations after renal transplantation. J Am Coll Surg 1997;184:63–9.

[37] Bobak DA. Gastrointestinal infections caused by cytomegalovirus. Curr Infect Dis Rep 2003;5:101–7.

[38] Lee CJ, Lian JD, Chang SW, et al. Lethal cytomegalovirus ischemic colitis presenting with fever of unknown origin. Transplant Infect Dis 2004;6:124–8.

[39] Koneru B, Selby R, O'Hair DP, et al. Nonobstructing colonic dilatation and colon perforations following renal transplantation. Arch Surg 1990;125:610–3.

[40] Scott TR, Graham SM, Schweitzer EJ, et al. Colonic necrosis following sodium polystyrene sulfonate (Kayexalate)–sorbitol enema in a renal transplant patient. Report of a case and review of the literature. Dis Colon Rectum 1993;36:607–9.

[41] Gerstman BB, Kirkman R, Platt R. Intestinal necrosis associated with postoperative orally administered sodium polystyrene sulfonate in sorbitol. Am J Kidney Dis 1992;20:159–61.

[42] McCune TR, Nylander WA, Van Buren DH, et al. Colonic screening prior to renal transplantation and its impact on post-transplant colonic complications. Clin Transplant 1992; 6:91–6.

[43] Lederman ED, McCoy G, Conti DJ, et al. Diverticulitis and polycystic kidney disease. Am Surg 2000;66:200–3.

[44] Stratta RJ. Clinical patterns and treatment of cytomegalovirus infection after solid-organ transplantation. Transplant Proc 1993;25(S):15–21.

[45] Snydman DR. Infection in solid organ transplantation. Transplant Infect Dis 1999;1:21–8.

[46] Rubin RH. Impact of cytomegalovirus infection on organ transplant recipients. Rev Infect Dis 1990;12(S):S754–66.

[47] Paya C, Humar A, Dominguez E, et al. Efficacy and safety of valganciclovir vs. oral ganciclovir for prevention of cytomegalovirus disease in solid organ transplant recipients. Am J Transplant 2004;4:611–20.

[48] Slifkin M, Tempesti P, Poutsiaka DD, et al. Late and atypical cytomegalovirus disease in solid-organ transplant recipients. Clin Infect Dis 2001;33:62–8.

[49] Mosimann F, Cuenoud PF, Steinhauslin F, et al. Herpes simplex esophagitis after renal transplantation. Transplant Int 1994;7:79–82.

[50] Patterson JE. Epidemiology of fungal infections in solid organ transplant patients. Transplant Infect Dis 1999;1:229–36.

[51] Tran MQ, Gohh RY, Morrissey PE, et al. Cryptosporidium infection in renal transplant patients. Clin Nephrol 2005;63:305–9.

[52] Palau LA, Pankey GA. Strongyloides hyperinfection in a renal transplant recipient receiving cyclosporine: possible Strongyloides stercoralis transmission by kidney transplant. Am J Trop Med Hyg 1997;57:413–5.

[53] Sellin JH. The pathophysiology of diarrhea. Clin Transplant 2001;15(S):2–10.

[54] Keven K, Basu A, Re L, et al. Clostridium difficile colitis in patients after kidney and pancreas-kidney transplantation. Transplant Infect Dis 2004;6:10–4.

[55] Behrend M. Adverse gastrointestinal effects of mycophenolate mofetil: aetiology, incidence and management. Drug Saf 2001;24:645–63.

[56] Knoll GA, MacDonald I, Khan A, et al. Mycophenolate mofetil dose reduction and the risk of acute rejection after renal transplantation. J Am Soc Nephrol 2003;14:2381–6.

SURGICAL
CLINICS OF
NORTH AMERICA

ELSEVIER
SAUNDERS

Surg Clin N Am 86 (2006) 1207–1217

# Hepatobiliary Surgery: Lessons Learned from Live Donor Hepatectomy

David Elwood, MD,
James J. Pomposelli, MD, PhD*

*Division of Hepatobiliary Surgery and Liver Transplantation,
Lahey Clinic Medical Center, Burlington, MA 01805, USA*

The liver is a complex organ system that is involved in a variety of life-sustaining processes including protein, carbohydrate, and lipid metabolism; the production, storage, and delivery of bile; and serves as an important component of the immune system. The liver is unique in that rapid tissue regeneration occurs after resection or injury, and affords the surgeon the opportunity to safely remove up to 60% to 70% of the liver volume for treatment of cancer or for use as a live donor graft for transplantation [1].

The complex development of the liver and biliary system in utero results in multiple and complicated anatomic variations. An absolute knowledge of these anatomic variations with careful dissection and identification of structures at the time of surgery is required for the safe performance of any hepatobiliary operation. Because of the unforgiving nature of the liver's vascular supply and the biliary system, errors in technique or judgment can be disastrous to the patient, and can result in life-long disability or death. The hepatobiliary surgeon of today must be able to integrate a broadening array of radiologic and liver resection techniques that may improve patient safety and surgical outcome. Equally important is the ability to quickly recognize postoperative complications so that prompt intervention can be instituted. Positive outcome requires a balance between sound judgment, technical acumen, and attention to detail.

In this article, we review "state-of-the-art" hepatic imaging technology that has greatly improved surgical planning and safety for live donor liver transplantation and hepatic tumor resection. Experience with a variety of resectional techniques is reviewed, as they are now a part of the armamentarium

* Corresponding author.
*E-mail address:* james.j.pomposelli@lahey.org (J.J. Pomposelli).

0039-6109/06/$ - see front matter © 2006 Elsevier Inc. All rights reserved.
doi:10.1016/j.suc.2006.06.012                              *surgical.theclinics.com*

of the modern hepatobiliary surgeon. Finally, we consider lessons learned from a multidisciplinary approach in live donor liver transplantation that are directly applicable to any patient undergoing major hepatic resection.

## Innovative imaging technology

The most common imaging technologies used for surgical planning in hepatobiliary practice are computed axial tomography (CT scan) and MRI. Although the resolution and speed of scanners have improved dramatically over the last several decades, both technologies are deficient in that data pertaining to three-dimensional organs, such as the liver, are typically presented in a two-dimensional format. As a result, the surgeon must go through the intellectual exercise of performing virtual three-dimensional reconstruction when planning an operative procedure.

The recent development of advanced imaging software coupled with a high-speed, multiarray CT scanner has enabled radiologists to transform two-dimensional information into three-dimensional renderings (MeVis, Hepavision, Bremen Germany). Moreover, CT imaging using cholegraffin can precisely identify biliary anatomy, obviating the need for preoperative endoscopic retrograde cholangiopancreatography (ERCP), with its attendant risks. This allows the hepatobiliary surgeon to visualize the spatial relationships of the interior structures of the liver and perform "virtual resections" preoperatively. Moreover, accurate estimations of resected and residual liver volumes can be obtained from the images (Fig. 1).

High-quality three-dimensional imaging has been especially important in live donor liver transplantation, where graft size is critical in avoiding

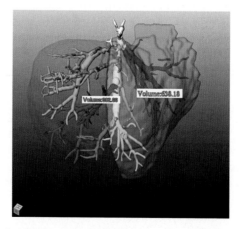

Fig. 1. Three-dimensional volumetric rendering of actual patient liver before live donation showing hepatic vein drainage. Each color represent individual segmental venous drainage. Volumes shown are for anatomic left and right lobes. In this case, a large accessory right hepatic vein (blue) drains directly into the vena cava.

"small-for-size" syndrome in recipients. Thus, donors with inadequate resectable liver graft volume can be identified preoperatively and noninvasively. During the postoperative period, three-dimensional and volumetric renderings have also been used to measure liver regeneration in both donors and recipients. This has provided a better understanding of the patterns of segmental hepatic growth in the donor and recipient, and it may help to elucidate the mechanism controlling liver regeneration. Increasingly, three-dimensional imaging technology is proving to be useful for planning complex procedures in a wide spectrum of surgical subspecialties including oncology (Fig. 2), urology, neurosurgery, reconstructive plastics, and vascular surgery.

## Technical aspects of live donor hepatectomy

Live donor liver transplantation has evolved from relatively small liver resections (left lateral segment) for transplantation in children [2], to anatomic left lobe grafts [3], and more recently, right lobe grafts [4]. Live donor hepatectomy is fundamentally different from hepatectomy for tumors in that the result must be a functional liver graft for the recipient and a viable residual liver in the donor. The donated graft requires adequate inflow with arterial and portal venous branches, as well as appropriate outflow with hepatic venous and biliary conduits. Meanwhile, the live donor surgeon must adhere to the dictum *primum non nocere* ("first, do no harm") when approaching the donor. The division of each conduit system must never

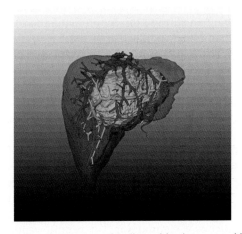

Fig. 2. Three-dimensional rendering of a patient liver with a large central hepatic mass demonstrating portal venous (green), arterial (red), and hepatic venous branches (blue). The tumor was resected with an extended left trisegmentectomy because posterior segments draining into the right hepatic vein could be saved.

compromise the donor remnant liver. Due to the inherent risk to the donor, the area of live donor liver transplantation has resulted in much ethical debate, but has been deemed acceptable after "research ethics consultation" [5]. Equally important is the concept of a multidisciplinary approach when initiating live donor programs to ensure that an adequate level of "field strength" is achieved by the team as eloquently described by the late Dr. Francis Moore in discussing the ethics of medical and surgical innovation [6]. The lessons learned from live donor liver transplantation contribute to the wealth of knowledge accumulated from liver resection for tumors, and may provide additional guidelines for the hepatobiliary surgeon.

Because donor hepatectomy is performed in an otherwise "healthy" individual, the impact of donor hepatectomy can be studied without the confounding variable-of-tumor burden or malnutrition. In this regard, the healthy live liver donor is an excellent model for studying postoperative complications, liver regeneration, and quality or life after major liver resection [7], and may be directly applicable to other patients undergoing liver surgery.

As mentioned previously, liver volume is an important determinant of postoperative outcome after major hepatic resection. In live donor liver transplantation, recipients should ideally receive a liver graft that has a volume of 0.8% to 1% of their body weight [8]. Because the largest liver graft obtained by right hepatic lobectomy is approximately 1000 g, recipients with body weights over 100 kg are generally not suitable recipients for live donor transplantation. Conversely, live liver donors left with less than 30% of their original liver volume are known to have higher morbidity rates, including prolonged periods of cholestasis and more infectious complications [9,10].

When performing hepatic resection for live donation, attention must be focused on performing an efficient dissection that adheres strictly to the predetermined plane, minimizes parenchymal destruction, and limits hemorrhage. Unlike liver resection for tumors, parenchymal division for live donation is performed without inflow occlusion, and must minimize ischemic insult and trauma to both the liver graft and the residual liver volume. Transection techniques that cause large zones of ischemic or traumatic "collateral damage" along the plane of division significantly decrease functional graft volume.

As with any hepatic resection, successful performance of a safe live donor hepatectomy requires the skillful and attentive participation from anesthesia staff. Routine use of central venous catheters for intraoperative monitoring and postoperative access as well as liberal use of epidural catheters for pain management have simplified management. Careful resuscitation of the patient while simultaneously maintaining low central venous pressures helps to minimize cut edge hemorrhage during hepatectomy. Actual blood loss between 300 to 700 mL is typical in our experience. Use of blood scavenging systems for reinfusion into the patient are routinely employed. Preoperative donation of 2 units of autologous blood separated into fresh frozen plasma and packed red blood cells has avoided the need for heterologous blood transfusion in our live donor experience.

Resection of the right lobe graft is approached through a "hockey-stick" right subcostal incision with a vertical extension to the xiphoid. We have abandoned the traditional bilateral subcostal "Chevron" or "Mercedes" incision. The subcostal incision is easier to close, less painful, and more cosmetic. There is a reduced incidence of incisional hernia.

After complete mobilization of the liver by dividing the falciform, right triangular, and coronary ligaments, the liver can be rotated to facilitate complete dissection of the retrohepatic vena cava. Not infrequently, a significant accessory hepatic vein ($\geq 5$ mm in diameter) drains the inferior posterior segment of the liver (segment VI) directly into the vena cava. This structure must be controlled during right hepatectomy for tumors, and it is preserved and reconstructed during live donation. It is important to carry out retrohepatic dissection of the vena cava up to the level of the hepatic veins, because this allows for direct visualization and safe division of the right hepatic vein and manual compression to control bleeding during parenchymal division.

Dissection of the porta hepatis is performed in a systematic fashion. All arterial and portal venous branches to the right lobe are dissected and surrounded with a vessel loop. Biliary dissection begins with a retrograde cholecystectomy. A probe is passed through the cystic duct stump into the hepatic duct to identify the right and left ducts to confirm biliary anatomy. Anatomic variations in the biliary tree are seen in up to 40% of all liver donors, and usually follow arterial and portal venous variations. Intraoperative findings of anatomy must be reconciled with preoperative imaging. If necessary, intraoperative cholangiography can be used. Precise determination of biliary anatomy helps to avoid iatrogenic injury and complications postoperatively [11].

The parenchymal transection is initiated after identifying the dissection plane between left and right lobes on the liver surface, and after mapping out the intrahepatic vascular structures. Temporary vascular inflow occlusion reveals Cantlie's line along which Glisson's capsule is scored with electrocautery. We use intraoperative ultrasound to trace the course of the middle hepatic vein from its origin between segments IV and V to its confluence with the vena cava. Larger branches draining the right lobe into the middle hepatic vein from segments V and VIII are identified and marked on the surface of the liver as a reminder as transection proceeds. In live donor liver transplantation, these branches need to be reconstructed in approximately 15% of cases [12]. Because donor safety is paramount in our program, we feel it is important to leave the middle hepatic vein with the donor. Some authors routinely take the middle hepatic vein with the graft to maximize venous drainage and graft size [13]. When performing parenchymal transection, it is important to realize that the middle hepatic vein does not lie directly posterior to the superficial line of demarcation on the capsule of the liver, but somewhat to the left. Thus, the line of transaction will not follow a flat sagittal plane, but will have a convex shape.

To keep the line of transaction on plane after the retrohepatic vena cava is dissected, we have adopted a modified sling suspension technique. A sterilized heavy shoelace is passed between the right and middle hepatic veins, under the liver, and up through the bifurcation of the left and right inflow vessels. The sling can be tightened and secured with clamps, elevating the liver away from the vena cava. In doing so, the shoelace serves as a plumb line to guide dissection, and it provides some control of venous bleeding by applying compression posterior to the liver. Additionally, the assisting surgeon can maintain manual control during transection by placing the left hand behind liver but just above the vena cava and elevating the liver. This maneuver protects the vena cava and left-sided vessels from injury and controls bleeding.

## Liver resection techniques

There are a myriad of instruments and techniques available for splitting the liver parenchyma. Most surgeons accomplish the transection using a "tissue fracture" or "finger fracture" technique. By gently crushing the parenchyma between two fingers or the tips of a small clamp, the softer tissues are pushed aside, exposing the vascular structures, which are then ligated and divided. This method is most effective and efficient at moving through tissue quickly, and it requires only several common instruments [14]. Finger or instrument fracturing serves well for most forms of hepatic resection; however, an unacceptably large volume of liver tissue is traumatized on either side of the split for use with the live donor procedure. The small hepatic vein branches are very fragile and tear easily, retracting into the parenchyma and causing hemorrhage. As the Pringle maneuver should be avoided during the live donor procedure, there can be a substantial amount of bleeding with this method until the split is completed. Consequently, there has been an impetus in live donor liver surgery to adopt novel techniques for performing parenchymal division.

A number of instruments have been marketed that use high-frequency vibrational energy to dissect tissue. Many have been applied to liver surgery with mixed results. The Harmonic Scalpel (Ethicon, Cincinnati, Ohio) is a set of ultrasonically activated shears. With blades vibrating at 55,500 Hertz, it collapses small blood vessels, forms a hemostatic coagulum of denatured protein, and divides tissue. The instrument has been used to dissect through liver parenchyma and expose underlying structures with minimal bleeding. However, beyond a depth of 2 to 3 cm, an alternative method must be employed to isolate and divide larger vessels and ducts. In our experience, the Harmonic Scalpel is effective but relatively slow. The Cavitron Ultrasonic Surgical Aspirator (CUSA, Valleylab, Boulder, Colorado) is an ultrasonically powered probe equipped with an aspirator. The oscillating tip selectively fragments parenchymal tissue sparing the vascular and ductal structures. The hand piece continuously irrigates and aspirates debris and blood away from the field, improving visibility. The bridging Glisson structures still need to be ligated, clipped, or electrocauterized. Bipolar electrocautery has been used in combination with CUSA to divide and seal the vessels and ducts. We have also found the CUSA effective but relatively slow for parenchymal transection. Failure to adequately occlude small fragile vessels and ducts leads to cut surface oozing and bile leakage. To prevent this phenomenon, dissecting and coagulating abilities are combined in the Dissecting Sealer (Tissuelink, Dover, New Hampshire). Saline solution is infused through the tip of the dissecting probe to couple radiofrequency energy to the tissue. This simultaneously precoagulates and divides parenchyma and small vessels. The tissue surface temperatures approach 100°C, far lower than that with traditional electrocautery. This prevents tissue burning, eschar, and smoke production. Although this technique has a theoretic advantages in patients with tumor because an additional several millimeters of margin is achieved, in our liver donor experience, the lost tissue volume along the resection plane proved to be prohibitive.

Our preferred instrument for transecting the parenchyma during live donor hepatectomy is the Helix Hydrojet (Erbe, Tubingen, Germany). With this device, a high-intensity pulsatile jet of saline blasts away the friable elements of the hepatic parenchyma, such as hepatocytes and adipose, preserving vascular structures and ducts. The hand piece also serves as a suction tip, clearing away fragments of tissue and blood. It is possible to achieve a very uniform and narrow plane of dissection. Small bridging structures are easily visualized. The Hydrojet even allows the surgeon to clean off major venous branches to facilitate clamping and ligation or to allow preservation. Pressure in the jet can be adjusted up to 50 kg/cm² to match the density of the liver tissue. Despite this substantial dissecting power, however, the Hydrojet has been found to have limited usefulness in the cirrhotic liver [15]. Also, we have found that parenchymal division time is perhaps slightly increased initially when using the Hydrojet. However, when compared with fracturing techniques, the blood loss has been significantly less. This benefit of reduced blood loss far outweighs the drawback of a longer dissection time in the live donor.

Regardless of the resection technique used, the cut surface along the transection plane invariably oozes blood and serum. We have found that this type of bleeding can be effectively controlled with the Argon Beam Coagulator (ABC, Valley Lab, Boulder, Colorado). This instrument emits a coaxial flow of Argon, and produces an electrocoagulation arc at the point of tissue touched by the stream. The inert Argon gas displaces oxygen at the site of cautery, limiting the amount of tissue that becomes carbonized [16]. Coagulation necrosis extends no deeper than 2.5 mm. The blowing effect of the Argon stream clears blood away from the target tissue, allowing for very effective coagulation to occur directly on the surfaces of the divided venous branches.

Once splitting of the liver is complete, the right hepatic artery and portal vein are clamped and divided in sequence. In a standard right hepatic resection for tumor, we employ an Endo-GIA stapler with vascular load (Ethicon, New Brunswick, New Jersey) to divide the right hepatic vein [17]. In the donor procedure, it is necessary to preserve as much extra-parenchymal vein length as possible; therefore, the right hepatic vein is divided sharply over a straight-blade vascular clamp. This maneuver is useful in situations where a stapler would not guarantee an adequate tumor margin or in the event that there is mass effect obstructing proper positioning of the stapler.

The question of whether or not to drain the cut edge of the liver after major resection is a contentious one. Detractors question the utility of draining [18] and cite reports associating drains with prolonged hospital stays and increased risks of infection after liver resection [19]. In one randomized study of 81 patients undergoing elective hepatic resection with and without drainage there was a significantly higher incidence of infected intraabdominal collections in the patients with drains [20]. Proponents site studies that suggest benefit with draining, because it allows earlier diagnosis of postoperative hemorrhage or bile leak [21]. By this strategy, draining is both diagnostic and therapeutic in being able to drain the leak until it seals over. It is our practice with the adult liver donors and all right hepatectomy patients to place a single Jackson Pratt drain for the purpose of monitoring postoperative bleeding and bile leakage. The drains are removed on postoperative day number 4 if there is no obvious biliary fistula.

Finally, any discussion of liver resectional surgery must now include mention of newer laparoscopic approaches. A number of centers in the United States, Europe, and Asia have reported laparoscopic lobar hepatectomies, segmentectomies, and nonanatomic resections with convincing results [22,23]. Laparoscopy reduces liver manipulation and diminishes the degree of wound morbidity postoperatively. In an attempt to extend this surgical innovation to liver transplant surgery, there have been several reports of laparoscopic donor left lateral hepatectomies in porcine models and in children [24,25]. These studies demonstrated the feasibility of current technology and methods to produce grafts without the use of vascular inflow occlusion, and to provide adequate vascular and ductal conduits [25]. For the time being, laparoscopic liver resection requires an advanced and specialized level of laparoscopic skills limited to a few centers. However, as these techniques are refined they are certain to be more widely applied to tumor resection and live donor surgery.

## Postoperative care

Because donor hepatectomy is performed in an otherwise "healthy" individual, the impact of donor hepatectomy can be studied without the confounding variable of tumor burden or malnutrition. In this regard, the healthy live liver donor is an excellent model for studying postoperative complications, liver regeneration, and quality or life after major liver resection [7], and may be directly applicable to other patients undergoing liver surgery.

The postoperative management of the live liver donor patients largely parallels that of other patients undergoing major hepatic resections. Several important differences between these two populations, however, have become apparent. The first is the increased level of pain that is experienced by these individuals. Donor patients have been shown to have significantly more pain than right lobe tumor resection patients [26]. In one comparative study, the donor group had higher postoperative pain scores, and the patients were 2.76 times more likely to have pain than those patients in the tumor resection group [26]. Maximal regional analgesia with thoracic epidural infusion catheters benefit these patients, allowing them to sleep adequately and participate in incentive spirometry and physical therapy. Despite the transient clotting function abnormalities that liver resection patients demonstrate, epidural catheters for analgesia are safe and effective [27]. Because it is our routine practice to obtain 2 units of autologous blood before live donor hepatectomy, 2 units of donor autologous fresh frozen plasma are available to correct clotting abnormalities for epidural catheter removal if required.

Second, unlike resection patients with tumors, donor patients typically complain of a profound malaise and nausea early in the postoperative period. This usually begins on the second or third day after surgery, but rarely lasts longer than 5 days. It is felt that these symptoms may reflect the fact that these individuals suddenly loose over half of their functional hepatic reserve. In contrast, patients undergoing hepatectomy for tumors, for example, lose much less functional liver and may have developed compensatory hypertrophy in the contralateral segments before surgery.

Both donors and recipients demonstrate rapid liver regeneration in the liver remnant immediately after surgery [1,28]. Exponential growth (regeneration) over the first 3 months continues, albeit at a much slower rate, for a full year postoperatively [1]. During this rapid growth phase, the substrate for regeneration is obtained from skeletal and visceral protein breakdown if exogenous nutrition support is not provided. For this reason, it has been our practice to begin nutrition support in the form of enteral nutrition or total parental nutrition (TPN) in the immediate postoperative period for all of the donors [9,29]. Because many donors are intolerant to enteral intake because of malaise and nausea, TPN helps to serve as a bridge to meet protein and caloric requirements until their oral intake is sufficient.

One metabolic derangement that commonly occurs after live donor right hepatectomy is the development of profound hypophosphatemia [29,30]. In our experience, the nadir of serum phosphate levels occurs at postoperative day 2 or 3, with 70% of donors developing serum phosphate levels below 1.0 mg/dL [29]. At that level, hypophosphatemia can be associated with cardiac dysfunction, hypoventilation, and impaired immunity. By aggressively repleting serum phosphate, profound hypophosphatemia can be avoided in most patients, reducing the risk of donor morbidity.

## Summary

Live donor liver transplantation is a surgical innovation that has proven to be a viable option for patients with end-staged liver disease. Improvements in preoperative imaging, surgical technique, and postoperative care contribute to favorable outcomes for both donors and recipients. These advances are also being applied more broadly to hepatic surgery. Novel three-dimensional modeling of the liver, which now includes the biliary system as well as the vascular structures, allows for precise planning of complex donor hepatectomies and oncologic resections. The instruments and techniques available to the modern day hepatobiliary surgeon help to limit hemorrhage during liver transaction and avoid the need for inflow hepatic occlusion, while allowing for more precise parenchymal dissection. Of course, the choice of tools and approach will always depend on the clinical situation, equipment availability, and above all, surgeon experience. The reciprocal relationship between the surgical advances in the fields of liver transplant surgery and hepatobiliary surgery over the past 2 decades have successfully reduced the morality of major liver resections to less than 5%.

## References

[1] Pomfret EA, Pomposelli JJ, Gordon FD, et al. Liver regeneration and surgical outcome in donors of right-lobe liver grafts. Transplantation 2003;76(1):5–10.

[2] Broelsch CE, Whitington PF, Emond JC, et al. Liver transplantation in children from living related donors. Surgical techniques and results. Ann Surg 1991;214(4):428–37 [discussion 37–9].

[3] Yamaoka Y, Tanaka K, Ozawa K. Liver transplantation from living-related donors. Clin Transpl 1993:179–83.

[4] Wachs ME, Bak TE, Karrer FM, et al. Adult living donor liver transplantation using a right hepatic lobe. Transplantation 1998;66(10):1313–6.

[5] Singer PA, Siegler M, Lantos JD, et al. The ethical assessment of innovative therapies: liver transplantation using living donors. Theor Med 1990;11(2):87–94.

[6] Moore FD. Therapeutic innovation: ethical boundaries in the initial clinical trials of new drugs and surgical procedures. CA Cancer J Clin 1970;20(4):212–27.

[7] Verbesey JE, Simpson MA, Pomposelli JJ, et al. Living donor adult liver transplantation: a longitudinal study of the donor's quality of life. Am J Transplant 2005;5(11): 2770–7.

[8] Inomata Y, Uemoto S, Asonuma K, et al. Right lobe graft in living donor liver transplantation. Transplantation 2000;69(2):258–64.

[9] Fan ST, Lo CM, Liu CL, et al. Safety of donors in live donor liver transplantation using right lobe grafts. Arch Surg 2000;135(3):336–40.

[10] Marcos A, Ham JM, Fisher RA, et al. Single-center analysis of the first 40 adult-to-adult living donor liver transplants using the right lobe. Liver Transpl 2000;6(3):296–301.

[11] Huang TL, Cheng YF, Chen CL, et al. Variants of the bile ducts: clinical application in the potential donor of living-related hepatic transplantation. Transplant Proc 1996;28(3): 1669–70.

[12] Pomposelli JJ, Verbesey J, Simpson MA, et al. Improved survival after live donor adult liver transplantation (LDALT) using right lobe grafts: program experience and lessons learned. Am J Transplant 2006;6(3):589–98.

[13] Fan ST, Lo CM, Liu CL, et al. Safety and necessity of including the middle hepatic vein in the right lobe graft in adult-to-adult live donor liver transplantation. Ann Surg 2003;238(1): 137–48.

[14] Lesurtel M, Selzner M, Petrowsky H, et al. How should transection of the liver be performed? A prospective randomized study in 100 consecutive patients: comparing four different transection strategies. Ann Surg 2005;242(6):814–22 [discussion 22–3].

[15] Une Y, Uchino J, Shimamura T, et al. Water jet scalpel for liver resection in hepatocellular carcinoma with or without cirrhosis. Int Surg 1996;81(1):45–8.

[16] Postema RR, ten Kate FJ, Terpstra OT. Less hepatic tissue necrosis after argon beam coagulation than after conventional electrocoagulation. Surg Gynecol Obstet 1993;176(2): 177–80.

[17] Fong Y, Blumgart LH. Useful stapling techniques in liver surgery. J Am Coll Surg 1997; 185(1):93–100.

[18] Liu CL, Fan ST, Lo CM, et al. Safety of donor right hepatectomy without abdominal drainage: a prospective evaluation in 100 consecutive liver donors. Liver Transpl 2005;11(3): 314–9.

[19] Fong Y, Brennan MF, Brown K, et al. Drainage is unnecessary after elective liver resection. Am J Surg 1996;171(1):158–62.

[20] Belghiti J, Kabbej M, Sauvanet A, et al. Drainage after elective hepatic resection. A randomized trial. Ann Surg 1993;218(6):748–53.

[21] Bona S, Gavelli A, Huguet C. The role of abdominal drainage after major hepatic resection. Am J Surg 1994;167(6):593–5.

[22] Mala T, Edwin B, Rosseland AR, et al. Laparoscopic liver resection: experience of 53 procedures at a single center. J Hepatobiliary Pancreat Surg 2005;12(4):298–303.

[23] O'Rourke N, Fielding G. Laparoscopic right hepatectomy: surgical technique. J Gastrointest Surg 2004;8(2):213–6.

[24] Kurian MS, Gagner M, Murakami Y, et al. Hand-assisted laparoscopic donor hepatectomy for living related transplantation in the porcine model. Surg Laparosc Endosc Percutan Tech 2002;12(4):232–7.

[25] Cherqui D, Soubrane O, Husson E, et al. Laparoscopic living donor hepatectomy for liver transplantation in children. Lancet 2002;359(9304):392–6.

[26] Cywinski JB, Parker BM, Xu M, et al. A comparison of postoperative pain control in patients after right lobe donor hepatectomy and major hepatic resection for tumor. Anesth Analg 2004;99(6):1747–52.

[27] Borromeo CJ, Stix MS, Lally A, et al. Epidural catheter and increased prothrombin time after right lobe hepatectomy for living donor transplantation. Anesth Analg 2000;91(5): 1139–41.

[28] Pomposelli JJ, Verbessey J, Simpson MA, et al. Improved survival after live donor adult liver transplantation (LDALT) using right lobe grafts: program experience and lessons learned. Am J Transplant 2006.

[29] Pomposelli JJ, Pomfret EA, Burns DL, et al. Life-threatening hypophosphatemia after right hepatic lobectomy for live donor adult liver transplantation. Liver Transpl 2001;7(7):637–42.

[30] Burak KW, Rosen CB, Fidler JL, et al. Hypophosphatemia after right hepatectomy for living donor liver transplantation. Can J Gastroenterol 2004;18(12):729–33.

ELSEVIER
SAUNDERS

SURGICAL
CLINICS OF
NORTH AMERICA

Surg Clin N Am 86 (2006) 1219–1235

# Living Kidney Donation: Evolution and Technical Aspects of Donor Nephrectomy

Paul E. Morrissey, MD[a],*, Anthony P. Monaco, MD[b]

[a]Brown Medical School, Rhode Island Hospital, 593 Eddy Street, Providence RI 02903, USA
[b]Harvard Medical School, Beth-Israel Deaconess Medical Center, One Deaconess Road,
Boston, MA 02215, USA

The first successful solid organ transplant was performed between 23-year-old identical twins in 1954. Joseph Murray, at the then Peter Bent Brigham Hospital in Boston, transplanted a healthy kidney from Ronald Herrick into his twin brother, Richard, who had end-stage renal disease as a result of chronic nephritis. Richard Herrick recovered uneventfully, married, and went on to live an active life, dying eight years later from causes unrelated to the transplant. Since that time, many thousands of patients have received successful transplants from living donors, whose evaluation and surgical care are the responsibility of the center or hospital doing the transplant—unlike deceased donor transplantation, which is administered by United Network for Organ Sharing (UNOS) through the coordinated efforts of 58 affiliated organ procurement organizations. Currently, in the United States, more than 6000 live donor kidney transplants are performed each year. In 2001, for the first time, there were more living organ donors in the United States than deceased organ donors.

Kidney transplantation from a live organ donor is recognized as an ethically acceptable practice. Nonetheless, this treatment affects not only the patient who has renal failure, but also the healthy person who volunteers to donate and whose interests are equally important. Although the risk of organ donation is considered to be acceptable, it is uniformly recognized that there are short- and long-term risks associated with living organ donation. The estimated operative mortality from living kidney donation ranges from 2 to 3 deaths per 10,000 cases. Even the first successful live donor renal transplant was nearly marred by a donor misadventure. While the attention

* Corresponding author.
*E-mail address:* pmorrissey@lifespan.org (P.E. Morrissey).

0039-6109/06/$ - see front matter © 2006 Elsevier Inc. All rights reserved.
doi:10.1016/j.suc.2006.06.008
*surgical.theclinics.com*

of those present focused on the recipient, the vascular clamp on the short arterial stump of the donor slipped off; the surgeon was fortunately able to control the brisk bleeding deep in the incision [1]. Tom Starzl, pioneer of liver transplantation, bemoaned the necessity of subjecting a healthy individual to the risks of surgery for the benefit of the affected recipient. He redoubled his concerns after a kidney donor under his care, who happened to be an athlete, required lower limb amputation because of complications arising from donor nephrectomy. Concerns over the welfare of the donor led early practitioners to question the ethical basis of living organ donation [2].

Living donation offers an alternative for individuals awaiting transplantation and increases the existing organ supply. At many centers, approximately 50% of the kidney transplants performed are from live donors. Living organ donation imparts numerous advantages (ie, reduced waiting time, prompt organ function, excellent allograft quality, less injury from cold storage) and one significant disadvantage—the requirement for a healthy individual to accept the risks of major surgical intervention for no direct medical benefit. Nonetheless, there are obvious psychological benefits for the donor, and the requisite expertise assures that the medical risk is sufficiently low as to justify living donation. Only kidney transplantation—and, to some extent, liver transplantation (addressed in a separate chapter)—are performed with any frequency (>50 cases per year in the United States); this article is limited to a discussion of kidney donation and technical aspects of the donor surgery.

## Qualifications for living donors

To qualify as a living donor, an individual must be in good general health and free from diabetes, cancer, active infection, and kidney disease. Individuals considered for living donation are usually between 18 and 70 years of age, but there is no absolute upper age limit, and adolescent donors have been used in exceptional cases. Gender and race are not factors in determining a successful match, but they do influence the quality of the allograft and might impact on long-term function. The living donor must first undergo a blood test to determine blood type compatibility with the recipient and an immunologic cross-match test to verify the absence of pre-formed anti-HLA antibodies to donor-specific antigens. If the donor and recipient have compatible (but not necessarily identical) blood types, the donor undergoes a medical history review and a complete physical examination. In addition (and typically before cross-match testing), ABO-compatible potential donors are evaluated by psychological testing, serum chemistries, serology, measurement of glomerular filtration rate (GFR), urinalysis, chest radiograph, and an electrocardiogram. Various guidelines for living kidney donor evaluation outline these criteria in greater detail [3].

## Consent for organ donation

A potential live organ donor should be competent, willing to donate, free of coercion, medically and psychosocially suitable, fully informed of the risks and benefits as a donor, and fully informed of the risks, benefits, and alternative treatment available to the recipient. Donors should not be called upon to donate in clinically hopeless situations; thus, the benefits to both donor and recipient must outweigh the risks associated with the donation and transplantation of the living donor organ [4]. Initially, living kidney transplantation was limited to only blood relatives, the practice justified on the basis that improved histocompatibility achieved with consanguineous donor–recipient combinations reduced recipient immunosuppression requirements and thereby reduced associated morbidity and mortality while achieving improved allograft survival. Recent advances in immunosuppressive therapy have now permitted highly successful kidney allograft survival rates in non-related (non-consanguineous) donor–recipient combinations (using spouses, friends, lovers, and even unacquainted, anonymous, non-directed donors). Thus, the requirement for consanguinity between living donors and recipients is no longer ethically required. The relationship between the donor and recipient should not alter the level of acceptable risk. Altruism has been the foundation of live organ donation since its inception. Strangers or non-directed, anonymous donors are increasingly common, and these donors share the same medical risks as related donors. Conversely, a familial relationship does not impose upon the donor (or the recipient) the necessity to take on additional medical risk to accomplish donation. In some circumstances, a familial bond might result in an undercurrent of coercion that does not exist in donation between strangers.

The consent for living donation should include a description of the surgical procedure and recuperative period, alternative donation procedures (even if only available at other transplant centers), the potential surgical complications for the donor, the medical uncertainties (including the potential for long-term donor complications), expected outcome of transplantation for the recipient, and transplant center-specific statistics of donor and recipient outcome. The disclosure process should permit a "cooling off period" between consent and the scheduled donor operation to provide the potential donor ample time to reconsider the decision to donate. It should be made clear to the donor that they are free not to donate, and some individual in the evaluation process should serve as an independent, confidential resource for the potential donor to express hesitations, concerns, or health problems that the donor might not wish to disclose in the presence of a family member. It is possible for negative psychological consequences to result from living donation. Living donors might feel pressured by their families into donating an organ and guilty if they are reluctant to go through with the procedure. Feelings of resentment might also occur if the recipient rejects the donated organ. Living donors must be made aware of the physical and psychological risks involved before they consent to donate an organ. Potential donors should be encouraged to discuss their feelings and concerns with a transplant professional, social worker, or other informed advocate.

## Preoperative imaging

The kidney is a mesodermal organ that develops from the metanephros, which appears in the fifth week of gestation and begins to function (make urine) about 6 weeks later [5]. The kidney originates in the pelvis and ascends to its retroperitoneal position overlying the psoas muscle. Variation in the number of renal arteries or veins is common; 20% to 25% of people have two or more vessels to a single kidney. Vascular variations arise from persistence of embryonic vessels that fail to degenerate when the definitive renal arteries form. Persistent blood supplies from the pelvis (iliac artery) and infrarenal aorta to the lower pole of the kidney are frequently observed. Division of the metanephric diverticulum (ureteric bud) can result in duplicated (or more commonly partially duplicated) renal pelvis or ureter that might influence the choice of kidney for procurement (Fig. 1).

Suitable donors undergo an arteriogram by way of femoral puncture, computerized tomographic angiography (CTA) or magnetic resonance angiography (MRA) to evaluate the kidney, ureter, and vascular supply. These tests visualize the renal artery and vein accurately as well as ureters and surrounding structures. CTA or MRA are preferred by most centers over

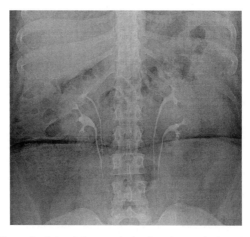

Fig. 1. A plain radiograph of the abdomen obtained at the conclusion of computerized tomographic angiography (CTA) demonstrates bilateral duplicated ureters in this kidney donor. The left kidney was procured by way of a mini-open donor nephrectomy. The two ureters were spatulated and anastomosed as a single entity with absorbable suture. The common end was implanted as a single ureteroneocystostomy.

formal arteriography, which is uncomfortable, cumbersome, and more inconvenient for the donor. The renal vasculature is accurately imaged with either CTA or MRA. Three-dimensional reconstructions contribute to the sensitivity of these studies (Fig. 2). Selection of which kidney to remove for donation is governed by several characteristics. Single vessels are preferred over multiple vessels, the larger of two normal kidneys is usually left in the donor, and kidneys with unilateral anomalies or minor pathology (eg, single cysts) are usually taken as donor organs. Everything else being equal, the left kidney is preferred for organ donation because of the longer left renal vein.

## Surgical procedure of living kidney donation

Traditionally, donor nephrectomy was performed through a 15 to 25 cm flank incision overlying the eleventh rib. Often, a portion of the rib was resected to assist with exposure. This approach was derived from urologic practice, where many of the surgeries are performed for cancer. Since its introduction in 1995 laparoscopic donor nephrectomy (LDN) has gained widespread acceptance, and currently one-half of all donor nephrectomies in the United States are accomplished by this technique. LDN boasted a shorter length of stay, decreased post-operative pain, and improved cosmetic results. As in many other areas of surgery, the availability of a new technology resulted in modifications of existing practices to adapt them to a new set of expectations. Nephrectomy by way of flank incision was replaced by several techniques of mini-open nephrectomy performed through

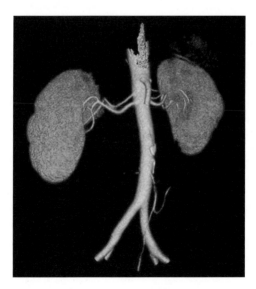

Fig. 2. A three-dimensional reconstruction of a CTA demonstrates two renal arteries on the right and tree renal arteries, including a small upper pole branch to the left kidney.

a 6 to 10 cm incision. Various retroperitoneal approaches were described, including a posterior approach and anterior approaches by way of transverse and longitudinal incisions.

## Technique of LDN

The technique for LDN was described in 1995 and pioneered in Baltimore at Johns Hopkins Medical Center and the University of Maryland. Only 5 years before, surgeons at Johns Hopkins performed the first laparoscopic nephrectomy to remove a diseased kidney. The minimally invasive procedure represented such an advance over nephrectomy by flank incision that it became accepted based on a few single-center reports and presentations at professional meetings. Hospitals across the country added the technique to their surgical repertoire despite a paucity of randomized, controlled trials [6,7]. Patients were offered the advantages of less pain, a shorter hospital stay, and quicker recovery. In addition, when the kidney was removed through a Pfannenstiel incision, the result was cosmetically superior.

The laparoscopic procedure was initially (and is typically) performed by way of a transabdominal approach either by pure laparoscopic (LDN) or hand-assisted (HADN) laparoscopic donor nephrectomy techniques. These two techniques differ in the timing and possible location of the incision for removal of the kidney. Without hand-assist the incision for kidney extraction is not made until the kidney is completely mobilized. Immediately before division of the renal vessels a 7 to 10 cm abdominal incision, commonly lower midline or Pfannenstiel, is created for retrieval of the kidney. The free kidney is withdrawn from the abdomen by hand or with a 15-mm endocatch device (retrieval bag) inserted through a port placed in the abdominal or suprapubic incision. The kidney can also be extracted through a left lower quadrant incision. Some surgeons prefer an upper quadrant transverse incision on the right side [8]. With the hand-assisted transabdominal procedure, a hand port is placed early in the surgery, usually by way of a midline incision, and a hand is used throughout for dissection, palpation, and retraction. Advocates of HADN point out the improved safety provided by immediate access to the renal hilum and great vessels in the setting of vascular injury and massive bleeding.

Laparoscopic donor nephrectomy can also be accomplished through a retroperitoneal approach, though far fewer cases have been reported. As with the transabdominal approach, this approach can be accomplished with a predominantly laparoscopic technique [9] or with a hand-assisted retroperitoneal method [10]. Blunt finger dissection of the peritoneum is followed by insufflation and trochar placement under direct vision. Once the operating environment has been established, the procedure is similar to a transabdominal approach minus the requirement to reflect the colon and spleen to expose the kidney.

The detailed procedure for laparoscopic donor nephrectomy is well described [11]. The preparation of the patient is the same as for open nephrectomy because the possibility of open conversion always exists. The patient is placed in a partial lateral decubitus position to allow for Pfannenstiel incision. The laparoscopic ports, generally three 10 to 12 mm ports, are placed in the left upper quadrant (left donor nephrectomy). A fourth working port (5 mm in size) is occasionally placed in the mid-axillary line for additional retraction. Pneumoperitoneum is established and laparoscopic exploration of the abdomen is undertaken. Because pneumoperitoneum decreases renal blood flow, vigorous hydration (4–6 L of crystalloid intravenously) is employed.

In brief, an incision is made along the line of Toldt and the colon from the splenic flexure to the proximal sigmoid region is reflected medially along with the spleen. The phrenocolic, lienorenal, and splenocolic ligaments are divided, as are the splenic attachments to the diaphragm (as necessary) to expose the anterior surface of the kidney, including the upper pole and hilum. Care is taken to leave the lateral retroperitoneal attachments of the kidney and Gerota's fascia intact. This action suspends the kidney and maintains favorable exposure of the renal vessels. The dissection involves three stages that can proceed in any sequence: mobilization of the ureter, isolation of the renal vessels (including division of all renal vein branches), and dissection of the superior pole of the kidney. Lastly, the kidney is freed completely by dividing the lateral and posterior attachments of Gerota's fascia. The ureter is isolated over the psoas muscle and mobilized inferiorly to the iliac vessels and superiorly to the renal hilum. Limited dissection of the ureter in the angle from the renal pelvis to the proximal ureter preserves its delicate blood supply. The gonadal vein is identified and traced to the renal vein, where it is divided between clips. The renal vein is freed from its adventitial attachments and the adrenal and lumbar veins are also clipped and divided. Two clips are placed on each side of the vessels; a right angle clip applier is often useful. The renal artery, which lies superior and posterior to the vein, is identified and freed by dividing the lymphatics and sympathetic nerve tissue with cautery (harmonic scalpel). The artery is exposed to its insertion at the aorta to achieve maximal length. Extensive distal dissection into the hilum is avoided to prevent injury to the branch vessels. Some authors advocate the application of topical papaverine to the renal artery because the retraction and dissection can induce vasospasm and restrict renal blood flow. Mobilizing the upper pole of the kidney is technically demanding. Care must be taken to avoid injury to the adrenal gland, spleen, upper pole of the kidney, and tail of the pancreas. The dissection in this area is often at the limits of standard instrumentation, camera visualization, and exposure. Having identified and isolated all of the critical structures for successful donation, the kidney can be mobilized completely by dividing the lateral and posterior attachments. If the mobilization was accomplished without hand-assist, an incision (midline, lower quadrant or Pfannenstiel) is made for extraction of the kidney, leaving the peritoneum intact. Pneumo-peritoneum is reestablished, systemic heparin sulfate is administered, and the ureter is divided after placing a 10 mm clip distally or using an endovas-cular gastrointestinal anastomosis (GIA) stapler. The kidney is retracted lat-erally within an endocatch retrieval bag, or by hand, and the vessels are divided (artery first) with the endovascular GIA stapler. The kidney is re-moved and flushed on a back table while the donor is inspected for meticu-lous hemostasis followed by closure of the incisions by any of several acceptable methods.

Warm ischemic time should be under 2 minutes. Initially many centers restricted LDN to left kidneys (described above) with normal arterial anat-omy; however, with growing experience right donor nephrectomies and do-nor nephrectomy in the setting of multiple renal arteries are commonly performed laparoscopically. Some centers prefer to recover the right kidney when vascular anomalies are present on the left kidney, accepting the shorter length of the right renal vein. Other centers prefer to recover the left kidney and reconstruct multiple vessels as required for implantation.

### Technical aspects of mini-open donor nephrectomy

A few centers modified open donor nephrectomy (ODN) in an attempt to achieve some of the benefits to the donor associated with LDN. There are several alternative approaches to ODN including those performed through a minimal flank incision, a dorsal lumbotomy incision, or an anterior retroper-itoneal approach. A Korean group developed a hybrid procedure of minila-parotomy that is performed with video assistance and the use of open and laparoscopic instrumentation [12]. The entire operation is performed through a 6 to 8 cm incision without trochars or pneumoperitoneum. The group de-signed a specialized set of piercing abdominal retractors that are introduced percutaneously and long-angled forceps to accomplish the procedure. They reported no ureteral complications and one case of delayed graft function (DGF) in 170 kidneys recovered by video-assisted minilaparotomy.

Shenoy and colleagues reported favorable results with an open posterior ap-proach accomplished through a 6 to 10 cm incision [13]. In 2002 Mital and col-leagues introduced "microinvasive donor nephrectomy," which resulted in an earlier return to diet, reduced length of stay, and decreased requirements for analgesics compared with published results for LDN [14]. In 2003 we modified our open donor operation after the technique of Mital and colleagues, per-forming all ODN through an anterior, retroperitoneal approach.

The anterior ODN is accomplished through an 8 to 10 cm incision (Fig. 3). The patient is placed in a semi-lateral decubitus position with a kid-ney rest and the operating table in 20° flexion. A transverse incision is extended from the tip of the eleventh rib to the border of the rectus mu-scle. Occasionally, adequate exposure requires that the incision be carried over the superior aspect of the eleventh rib for an additional 1 to 2 cm.

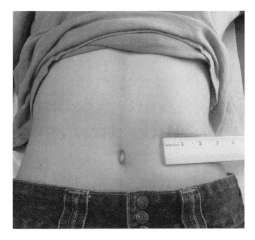

Fig. 3. Three weeks after mini-open donor nephrectomy, this patient has returned to college and routine physical activities. The 3-inch incision extends transversely from the tip of the eleventh rib to the border of the rectus abdominis muscle.

Alternatively, incising the rectus sheath followed by mobilization and retraction of the intact rectus abdominis muscle increases medial exposure and access to the renal hilum [15]. Rib resection is not required nor is elevation of the intercostal muscles with a periosteal elevator. Unlike the flank approach, the lung pleura are not proximate to the incision, eliminating the possibility of pneumothorax. The surgery is performed entirely retroperitoneally with dissection beginning over the psoas muscle toward the distal ureter. Overlying the kidney the peritoneum fuses with Gerota's fascia, making the retroperitoneal plane difficult to define; therefore, beginning the blunt dissection anterior to the ureter (caudal and lateral) is technically easier. The transversalis fascia is incised laterally, and gentle, blunt dissection is performed to make space for a hand-held retractor in the inferior aspect of the incision. The intermediate stratum of the retroperitoneal connective tissue is separated from the transversalis fascia, and the retroperitoneal space is further defined as the dissection continues cephalad. The peritoneum is retracted medially and exposure afforded by the Bookwalter or omnitract retractor. The ureter is mobilized from just above the iliac vessels to the renal hilum. Gerota's fascia is incised longitudinally along the lateral aspect of the kidney, and the kidney is mobilized by dividing the avascular attachments to the perinephric fat. Excess perinephric fat can be resected as required for optimal exposure through this small incision. The renal pedicle is exposed by developing the plane between the colon and its mesentery, and the retroperitoneal connective tissue overlying the kidney medially. Special care is taken to leave the perihilar fat intact and avoid dissection, and hence injury, to the branches of the main renal vessels within the hilum. Branches of the renal vein are divided between metal clips or sutures and the renal vessels are controlled with both suture ligatures and clips. The use of two nonabsorbable polymer ligating clips (Hemolock clip, Pilling Weck, Fort Lauderdale, Florida) appears to be adequate for controlling the vessels, although we continue to favor a transfixing suture in addition to a locking clip on the renal artery. The renal vein is divided below the adrenal branch and the renal artery divided 5 mm from the aorta. The ureter is clipped and divided 2 to 3 cm above the iliac bifurcation. After achieving hemostasis, bupivicaine (0.5%) is infiltrated along the mid-axillary line over ribs 10, 11, and 12 and along the length of the incision. Closure of the abdominal muscle layers (two layers) and skin is accomplished with absorbable sutures.

Post-operative management was the same for all three approaches. Favorable results using ketorolac for post-operative pain management were reported, although in the setting of major vascular surgery and iatrogenic renal insufficiency (albeit temporary) this drug might not intuitively seem a logical choice [16]. We incorporated its use in our postoperative regimen as a supplement to narcotic analgesia and observed less nausea and improved analgesia compared with narcotic agents. The patient is allowed clear liquids when awake and advanced to a regular diet at their discretion. The donor can begin eating often within hours of the procedure, particularly when the surgery is limited to the retroperitoneum. The Foley catheter is removed the morning after surgery and the patient is encouraged to ambulate. Patients are discharged to home 2 to 4 days after surgery. Some centers have discharged the donor after a single day, but it is unclear to what end this is encouraged.

### Results for donor nephrectomy at the Rhode Island Hospital

We have offered LDN since July 2000. Over this time period we continued to perform ODN with patients according to donor preference and the once-monthly availability of a laparoscopic surgeon. Over that time period 206 donor nephrectomies were performed including 82 from a traditional flank incision, 39 LDN, and 85 open cases through an anterior retroperitoneal approach (mini-ODN). Our results with mini-ODN have been described elsewhere and have been updated for this report [17]. LDN was performed with complete laparoscopic dissection and kidney retrieval by way of a Pfannenstiel incision. Open nephrectomies were performed by way of a 15 to 20 cm flank incision over the eleventh rib (July 2000 to September 2002) and by way of an 8 to 10 cm transverse incision from the tip of the eleventh rib to the border of the rectus muscle (October 2002 to December 2005).

There were no differences in donor age, gender, or relation to the recipient. Donor length of stay and narcotic requirements were significantly shorter for LDN as compared with traditional ODN; however, no significant differences were observed for length of stay (3.0 ± 0.9 days versus 3.3 ± 0.8 days) or narcotic requirements for LDN compared with mini-ODN. One patient after LDN and two patients following mini-ODN required oral narcotics beyond 1 week. The only difference noted between LDN and mini-ODN was the higher cost of laparoscopy, with the majority of the increase because of instrumentation. Wound complications included one case of flank bulge in the traditional ODN group and one wound infection after LDN. No patient required admission beyond 5 days in any group. There was one re-admission for treatment of an infected wound. One patient in the LDN group returned to the operating room to control bleeding from an epigastric artery injured during trochar placement. That patient and one in the traditional ODN group required blood transfusion. Minor complaints (numbness and transient hyperesthesia) caused by intercostal nerve trauma were common after ODN but resolved without intervention and did not result in prolonged morbidity. Two cases in the mini-ODN were complicated by primary graft nonfunction, one related to postoperative bleeding and another to prolonged warm ischemic time at the recipient operation; all other kidneys (204 of 206) functioned promptly after surgery. The recipient's renal function at 1 month and 1 year after transplantation was similar in all three groups. In summary, all three approaches resulted in a high rate of technical success and equivalent early and late renal function. Mini-ODN provided comparable donor benefits to LDN.

## Recovery after donor nephrectomy

A post-operative check-up follows in 2 to 4 weeks. In addition, UNOS recommends donor follow-up at 6 and 12 months after the surgery, at which time the function of the remaining kidney is assessed. As a result of hyperfiltration and modest glomerular hypertrophy, the remaining kidney ultimately achieves approximately 75% to 80% of the pre-donation glomerular filtration rate. After the 1-year visit most centers discharge donors with no ongoing issues to the care of their primary care physician with further follow-up at the transplant center on an as-needed basis. Some groups, particularly certain European centers, continue with indefinite yearly follow-up [18]. These reports and retrospective analyses of patients decades following nephrectomy confirm the long-term safety of uninephrectomy.

A living donor registry that would collect demographic, clinical, and outcome information on all living organ donors has been proposed for the United States. The rationale for the development of such a registry includes concern for donor well-being, limitations of current knowledge regarding the long-term consequences of donation, and the need within the transplantation community to develop mechanisms to provide for quality assurance assessments. Recently, there has been a movement to accept kidney donors that traditionally would have been excluded, including donors with a history of renal stones or gestational diabetes, medically-controlled high blood pressure, or obesity. As more centers accept these "high-risk" donors, the necessity for a critical review of their outcomes provides yet another reason to establish a donor registry.

There should be no change in a donor's ability to acquire life or health insurance after donor nephrectomy. There appears to be no higher likelihood of long-term consequences of kidney donation such as including hypertension and renal disease. In fact, some studies have shown an increased life expectancy after kidney donation, perhaps related to the selection process that excludes potential donors who have pre-existing medical illness. There are no direct medical costs for kidney donors or their insurers. The recipient's health insurance provides coverage for the donor's evaluation, work-up, surgery, and all necessary follow-up care. If the recipient is covered by a private insurance plan, most insurance companies pay 100% of the donor's expenses. If the recipient is covered by Medicare's end-stage renal disease program, Medicare Part A pays all of the donor's medical expenses including preliminary testing, the transplant operation, and postoperative recovery costs. Medicare Part B pays for physician services during the hospital stay. Medicare also covers follow-up care if complications arise following the donation. In the rare (but reported) instance that a previous donor develops end-stage renal disease, UNOS regulations provide a priority kidney allocation that virtually eliminates waiting time for a deceased donor kidney should the patient be a suitable candidate for transplantation.

## Comparative advantages and disadvantages of open (mini-ODN) versus LDN

LDN is now a widely accepted procedure. After the introduction of LDN in 1995, most surgeons adopted one of three strategies: (1) maintain the status quo (nephrectomy by flank incision), (2) change to LDN, or (3) modify the open approach by one of several less invasive ODN techniques. Open surgery offers several benefits including a simple retroperitoneal approach, which reduces the possibility of injury to the bowel, spleen, or other abdominal structures. It also reduces the risk of hernia and adhesions, it avoids pneumoperitoneum, possibly reducing renal injury (delayed graft function), it allows direct, open control of the renal vasculature, possibly enhancing donor safety, and it reduces operative time and cost. Surgeons who are skilled at nephrectomy but who have not developed advanced laparoscopic skills are able to safely continue the practice of donor nephrectomy.

The advantages of LDN for the donor are well documented; however, modest differences in hospital stay and narcotic requirements are minor in comparison to the possibility of compromised donor safety. The safety of LDN compared with ODN remains uncertain. Advanced laparoscopic techniques are unfamiliar to many transplant surgeons. Furthermore, there have been reports of significant complications, including a suggestion of a higher mortality with LDN [19,20]. Emergent conversions to an open operation, reoperation for post-operative bleeding, and several grave complications have been documented (Box 1). There is a suggestion that the benefits derived from laparoscopic donor nephrectomy are achieved at the price of a

**Box 1. Reported surgical complications following laparoscopic and open donor nephrectomy**

*Grave complications*
Death (two cases in 1999–2001 [19])
Fatal cerebral gas embolism
Persistent vegetative state (after massive hemorrhage)
Pulmonary embolism
Myocardial infarction
Major vascular injury
Renal vascular injury requiring transfusion
Venacaval injury
Trochar trauma (iliac artery, aorta)
Stapler malfunction
Splenic capsule tear, splenectomy
Liver laceration
Epigastric artery injury

*Gastrointestinal complications*
Small bowel perforation (thermal injury)
Colon injury
Serosal tear
Prolonged ileus
Bowel obstruction (hernia and adhesions)
Hernia (port site, internal, incisional)

*Lung complications*
Atelectasis
Pneumothorax
Pneumonia

*Miscellaneous*
Retained sponge
Adrenalectomy
Rhabdomyolysis
Deep venous thrombosis
Chylous ascites requiring prolonged parenteral nutrition (TPN)
Persistent abdominal pain
Wound infection
Nerve injury/neuropathy
Pneumonia
Post-operative fever and infection

*Transplanted kidney (recipient operation)*
Delayed graft function
Ureteral complications
Renovascular thrombosis

heightened donor operative risk. In contrast to ODN, the vast majority of LDNs are accomplished transperitoneally, which increases the likelihood of intra-abdominal organ injury and carries a life-long risk of hernia or bowel obstruction because of adhesions. LDN might predispose patients to acute tubular necrosis (ATN) caused by renal artery vasospasm during the dissection or as a consequence of pneumoperitoneum. For the recipient operation, higher rates of ATN, ureteral necrosis, and graft thrombosis have been reported [21]. Some complications are uniquely reported in the laparoscopic experience including vascular and enteric injury during trochar placement, port site hernia, thermal bowel injury, chylous ascites, and adverse effects of abdominal insufflation [22]. Some groups are reluctant to perform laparoscopic right nephrectomy because of concerns over vessel length. Many centers have opted to recover left kidneys with multiple renal arteries and perform a back-table reconstruction rather than procure a right kidney with normal vasculature. This practice further increases the technical demands of the recipient surgery.

HADN improves vascular control, might shorten operative times, and has been proposed as a safer alternative to LDN. HADN might offer advantages in complex or high-risk patients and facilitate teaching the procedure to residents and fellows. The benefit of hand-assist might be greater for transplant surgeons who do not routinely perform laparoscopic procedures. The primary disadvantage of HADN is the necessity of placing a hand port in a potentially more painful and less cosmetically desirable position compared with the Pfannenstiel incision used in LDN. No randomized trials have compared any of the LDN approaches with each other or with any of the mini-open techniques. Several single-center series have demonstrated the safety each of these approaches. For now, surgical experience and individual expertise should dictate the technique best suited for each transplant center or particular donor.

In summary, the accumulated literature suggests that the many modifications of the flank approach to nephrectomy for living donors are equivalent. Modified ODN (mini-ODN) shares the same advantages as LDN, namely, reduced requirement for analgesics, shorter length of stay, lower incidence of neuropathy, absence of flank bulge, and no risk of pneumothorax. Certainly LDN is not a panacea. The significant learning curve for the procedure is widely acknowledged. There is a long history of safety with ODN; the many reported complications of LDN suggest caution in adopting the procedure.

## Positive aspects of living donation

Living donation of any kind has several advantages over kidney transplantation with a deceased donor allograft. Living donation eliminates the recipient's need for placement on the national waiting list. This, in turn, results in reduced dialysis time and correlates with improved post-transplant survival [23]. Recipients who have pre-formed anti-HLA antibodies can undergo desensitization protocols that permit transplantation from donors to whom they exhibit positive antibody-mediated cross-matches; such protocols cannot be effectively used with deceased donor transplants [24]. Transplant surgery can be scheduled at a mutually agreed upon time rather than performed as an emergency operation. Because the operation can be scheduled in advance, the recipient can begin taking immunosuppressant drugs before the operation. The use of so-called marginal, extended criteria donors or donors after cardiac death is avoided. Transplants from living donors are also more successful because allograft injury from brain death, cold storage, and recovery is avoided or minimized, thereby achieving a greater functional nephron mass from the transplant. Similarly, avoidance of ischemia–reperfusion injury reduces up-regulation of allograft MHC antigens and reduced graft immunogenicity [25]. The higher rate of compatibility and reduced organ injury might decrease the risk of organ rejection. Perhaps the most important aspect of living donation is the ability to perform a pre-emptive renal transplant (before initiating dialysis) and the absence of exposure to a kidney with marginal function. The multiple advantages associated with living donor kidney transplants provide the basis for superior results versus deceased donor kidneys from every standpoint analyzed [26]. Finally, a less quantifiable, but no less profound psychological benefit is derived from living donor transplantation. The recipient can experience positive feelings knowing that the gift came from a loved one or a caring stranger. The donor experiences the satisfaction of knowing that he or she has contributed to the improved health of the recipient.

## Summary

Kidney transplantation has relied upon living donors since its inception. The number and percentage of kidney transplantations from a living donor source has increased every year over the past 20 years. Maintenance of the health and safety of the donor should be the transplant team's foremost concern. The transplant team (including a designated donor advocate) and the potential donor–recipient pair should determine if the benefits of the planned donation outweigh the risks. The risks of a complication to the live kidney donor should be minimized. Donor procedures should only be performed at centers and by surgeons with appropriate expertise.

LDN gained widespread popularity over the past decade. The rationale for adopting this procedure was the reduced pain and quicker recovery time compared with ODN. Two institutions introduced the procedure, which became widely adopted in the absence of randomized trials. Later in the experience, two randomized trials compared LDN with a traditional flank approach. These confirmed the more rapid recovery for the donor and the lack of inferiority for LDN in terms of recipient outcomes. Challenged by the considerable benefits of LDN over the traditional flank operation, surgeons in the transplant community developed several less invasive approaches to ODN. These newer procedures offered kidney donors a rapid recovery with acceptable risk. We, and others, have shown that the recovery benefits of mini-ODN, whether by lumbotomy or anterior retroperitoneal approach, are interchangeable with LDN.

Mini-ODN provides an open approach to donor nephrectomy that offers many advantages. It allows the surgeon who has a traditionally trained background to perform a safe, minimally invasive operation without laparoscopic technology. The operation is equally applicable to right or left nephrectomy. In fact, we have employed bilateral mini-ODN through 6 to 7 cm incisions to remove the native kidneys of patients who have end-stage renal disease. For the purpose of transplantation, ODN provides excellent length of the donor ureter, renal vein, and artery and avoidance of hemodynamic effects associated with pneumoperitoneum, which can adversely affect early allograft function. Open control of the renal vasculature might be safer. The comparable outcomes for donor convalescence make this procedure an attractive alternative to LDN.

## References

[1] Tilney NL. Transplant: from myth to reality. New Haven: Yale University Press; 2003.
[2] Merrill JP. Statement of the Committee on Morals and Ethics of the Transplantation Society. Ann Intern Med 1971;75:631–3.
[3] Davis CL. Evaluation of the living kidney donor: current perspectives. Am J Kidney Dis 2004;43:508–30.
[4] Abecassis M, Adams M, Adams P, et al. Consensus statement on the live organ donor. JAMA 2000;284:2919–26.
[5] Moore KL. Before we are born: basic embryology and birth defects. 3rd edition. Philadelphia: WB Saunders; 1989.
[6] Wolf JS, Merion RM, Leichtman AB, et al. Randomized controlled trial of hand-assisted laparoscopic versus open surgical live donor nephrectomy. Transplantation 2001;72:284–90.
[7] Tooher RL, Rao MM, Scott DF, et al. A systematic review of laparoscopic live-donor nephrectomy. Transplantation 2004;78:404–14.
[8] Ratner LE, Fabrizio M, Chavin K, et al. Technical considerations in the delivery of the kidney during laparoscopic live-donor nephrectomy. J Am Coll Surg 1999;189:427–30.
[9] Abbou CC, Rabii R, Hoznek A, et al. Nephrectomy in a living donor by retroperitoneal laparoscopy or lomboscopy. Ann Urol (Paris) 2000;34:312–8 [in French].
[10] Wadstrom J. Hand-assisted retroperitoneoscopic live donor nephrectomy: experience from the first 75 consecutive cases. Transplantation 2005;80:1060–6.
[11] Fabrizio MD. Laparoscopic live donor nephrectomy. In: Bishoff JT, Kavoussi LR, editors. Atlas of laparoscopic retroperitoneal surgery. New York: WB Saunders; 2000. p. 121–34.
[12] Kim SI, Rha KH, Lee JH. Favorable outcomes among recipients of living-donor nephrectomy using video-assisted minilaparotomy. Transplantation 2004;77:1725–8.
[13] Shenoy S, Lowell JA, Ramachandran V, et al. The ideal living donor nephrectomy "mini-nephrectomy" through a posterior transcostal approach. J Am Coll Surg 2002;194:240–6.
[14] Mital D, Coogan CL, Jensik SC. Microinvasive donor nephrectomy. Transplant Proc 2003; 35:835–7.
[15] Redman JF. An anterior extraperitoneal incision for donor nephrectomy that spares the rectus abdominis muscle and anterior abdominal wall nerves. J Urol 2000;164:1898–900.

[16] Freedland SJ, Blanco-Yarosh M, Sun JC, et al. Ketorolac-based analgesia improves outcomes for living kidney donors. Transplantation 2002;73(5):741–5.

[17] Morrissey PE, Gautam A, Amaral JF, et al. Keeping up with the Jones's: open donor nephrectomy in the laparoscopic era. Transplant Proc 2004;36:1285–7.

[18] Thiel GT, Nolte C, Tsinalis D. The Swiss Organ Living Donor Health Registry (SOL-DHR). Ther Umsch 2005;62:449–57 [in German].

[19] Matas AJ, Bartlett ST, Leichtman AB, et al. Morbidity and mortality after living kidney donation, 1999–2001: survey of United States transplant centers. Am J Transplant 2003;3: 830–4.

[20] Friedman Al, Ratner LE, Peters TG. Fatal and non-fatal hemorrhagic complications of living kidney donation [abstract]. Am J Transplant 2004;8:370.

[21] Bartlett ST. Laparoscopic donor nephrectomy after seven years. Am J Transplant 2002;2: 896–7.

[22] Tan HP, Shapiro R, Montgomery RA, et al. Proposed live donor nephrectomy complication classification scheme. Transplantation 2006;81:1221–3.

[23] Mange KC, Joffe MM, Feldman HI. Effect of the use or nonuse of long-term dialysis on the subsequent survival of renal transplants from living donors. N Engl J Med 2001;344:726–31.

[24] Montgomery RA, Zachary AA. Transplanting patients with a positive donor-specific crossmatch: a single center's perspective. Pediatr Trans 2004;8(6):535–42.

[25] Pratschke J, Kofla G, Wilhelm MJ, et al. Improvements in early behavior of rat kidney allografts after treatment of the brain-dead donor. Ann Surg 2001;234:732–40.

[26] Mandal AK, Snyder JJ, Gilbertson DT, et al. Does cadaveric donor renal transplantation ever provide better outcomes than live-donor renal transplantation? Transplantation 2003;75:494–500.

ELSEVIER
SAUNDERS

SURGICAL
CLINICS OF
NORTH AMERICA

Surg Clin N Am 86 (2006) 1237–1255

# Orthopedic Complications of Solid-Organ Transplantation

## Roy K. Aaron, MD*, Deborah McK. Ciombor, PhD

*Department of Orthopaedics, Brown Medical School, 100 Butler Drive,
Providence, RI 02906, USA*

Organ transplantation has undeniably increased the longevity and quality of life of patients with end-stage organ failure. However, it has introduced the skeletal complications of (1) fragility fractures and decreased bone density due to pre-transplant bone loss and immunosuppressive therapy, and (2) avascular necrosis leading to subchondral fracture and secondary osteoarthritis. This article reviews these two skeletal complications of solid organ transplantation that lead to structural failure of bone and result in significant morbidity and reduced quality of life.

### Bone mineral density and fractures

Measurement of bone mineral density is now the standard way of assessing structural bone composition with physiologic and clinical relevance. It can be accomplished with many techniques, including ultrasound, single and dual photon densitometry, quantitative CT, and dual energy X-ray absorptiometry (DEXA). If cost, radiation exposure, and precision are factored in, DEXA is the commonly preferred method. Three sites are typically screened: the forearm for cortical bone, the spine for trabecular bone, and the hip for a composite of cortical and trabecular bone. The Z-score compares bone mineral density to an age-, gender-, and ethnic group-matched cohort, while the T-score compares bone mineral density to peak bone mass for Caucasian females age 25 to 35. Scores are reported as mean ± standard deviation. If the scores are less than −1 standard deviation from the mean, the bone mineral density is normal. A bone mineral density −1 to −2 standard deviations from the mean is termed osteopenia. Bone mineral density greater than −2 standard deviations from the mean is

---

* Corresponding author.
  *E-mail address:* roy_aaron@brown.edu (R.K. Aaron).

*surgical.theclinics.com*

called osteoporosis. The terminology is unfortunate, because patients with osteomalacia, hyperparathyroidism, and other metabolic bone diseases, are included in the descriptors, and the use of this nomenclature should not be construed as specifying a particular histopathologic diagnosis. In the setting of organ transplantation, reduced bone mineral density and an elevated fracture risk are seen both pre- and posttransplantation, with a rapid decrease in bone mineral density observed in the immediate post-transplant period. The histologic hallmarks of osteoporosis are reduced bone volume; thin, sparse, and occasionally discontinuous trabeculae; and thin cortices with a concomitant increase in the marrow space (Fig. 1).

The decision for clinical intervention is often based solely on the hip T-score; however, consideration of risk factors for fractures should add another level of sophistication to clinical decision making. An individual's risk of fracture is multifactorial, and can be assessed from a combination of clinical risk factors and bone density. There is a general, inverse relationship between bone density and fracture risk. However, fracture risk is also related to muscle strength, balance, and propensity to fall. There are several ways to assess the risk of fracture in patients with low bone density. The National Osteoporosis Foundation has compiled a list of risk factors, including the presence of previous fracture, a first-degree relative with fracture, body weight of less than 127 pounds, current smoker, rheumatoid arthritis or celiac disease, corticosteroid intake, and high alcohol consumption. The Fracture Index uses bone mineral density, age, and clinical factors to assess fracture risk [1]. The probability of sustaining a fragility fracture due to osteoporosis can be estimated by age and T-score [2]. The risk of fracture can be reduced by simple alterations in an individual's physical environment, careful attention to

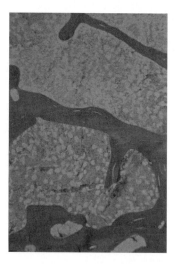

Fig. 1. Iliac crest biopsy of osteoporotic bone. Thin, delicate trabeculae are observed with marked reduction in trabecular volume.

medications, and physical training that improves balance and strength as well as therapeutic interventions to increase bone mineral density.

In patients with solid-organ transplantation, risk factors for fracture are related to decreased bone mineral density before transplantation and further loss of bone density occurring after transplantation. Bone loss and fracture in renal osteodystrophy and after renal transplantation are discussed separately. In patients with heart, lung, and liver transplants, fracture risk is related both to pretransplant bone loss associated with chronic disease and rapid bone loss after transplantation. Posttransplantation factors are related to immunosuppressive therapy and inactivity. The risk of fracture after cardiac transplantation has been reported to range from 6% to 21% [3–6]. Patients with chronic pulmonary disease undergoing lung transplantation have a particularly high risk of pretransplantation osteoporosis and fracture risk ranging from 10% to 30% [7,8]. Liver transplantation is also associated with an elevated risk of fractures, which has been reported to be 13% to 53% [6,9]. Fractures occur both in vertebral and long bones, and, although healing is the rule, treatment intervention is often required (Fig. 2). In addition to radiographically obvious fractures, stress fractures are common in solid-organ transplantations, and may be a source of bone pain that is inapparent on plain X-rays (Fig. 3). Stress fractures may require investigation with more sophisticated imaging techniques, either technetium bone scan or magnetic resonance imaging. A high index of suspicion for stress fractures should be maintained in the setting of chronic disease and organ transplantation. Although spontaneous healing of stress fractures is the rule, they may be a source of prolonged bone pain, disability, and, when in the lower

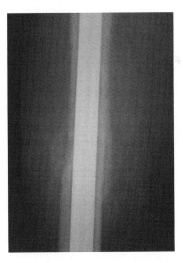

Fig. 2. Long bone fracture healing in renal osteodystrophy. The fracture has been internally fixed with an intramedullary rod. Callus formation can be seen around the fracture site. Although delay in fracture healing may be observed, eventual healing of well-stabilized fractures is expected.

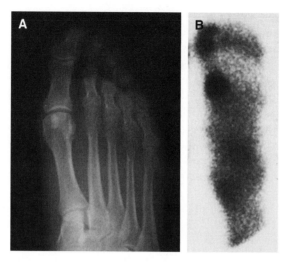

Fig. 3. Stress fracture. (*A*) Plain radiograph of the foot in which a stress fracture is inapparent. (*B*) $^{99}$Tc bone scan demonstrating uptake at a stress fracture site at the first metatarsal head.

extremities, impairment of gait, which may interfere with weight-bearing exercise and contribute further to loss of bone mineral.

Loss of bone density before transplantation (pretransplant bone disease) is present in heart, lung, and liver transplant patients, as well as in those with renal osteodystrophy and kidney transplantation. Malnutrition, decreased weight-bearing exercise, and medications contribute to pretransplant bone disease. Special features in the pathophysiology of end-stage organ diseases or associated treatment interventions may contribute to pretransplant bone disease. For example, in patients with chronic cardiac disease, loop diuretics can increase urinary calcium loss and have been associated with increased risk of fractures [10]. Anticoagulation therapy with warfarin has also been associated with increased fracture risk [11]. Many patients with chronic lung disease are treated with high doses of glucocorticoids before transplantation, and decreased bone mineral density and elevated risk of fragility fractures have been reported in this patient population [12,13]. Vertebral fractures have been reported to occur in approximately 25% of patients with chronic lung disease treated with glucocorticoids. Patients with chronic hepatic failure due to cholestatic disease, primary biliary cirrhosis, and primary sclerosing cholangitis have higher rates of osteoporosis and fragility fractures.

*Loss of bone mineral density after organ transplantation and the effects of immunosuppressive regimens*

In the first year after organ transplantation, bone mineral density declines substantially, up to 10%, although it appears to stabilize after the first year posttransplantation. There are several reasons for the loss of bone mineral density after transplantation, including the effects of chronic illness, lack of weight-bearing exercise, and the use of immunosuppressive regimens, notably the use of glucocorticoids. Reductions in bone mineral density and increased risk of fractures have been documented in patients undergoing cardiac transplantation. Fracture rates of 15% to 30% have been reported, mostly involving the vertebral body [6,14]. Decreases in bone mineral density and an elevated fracture risk are seen in patients with lung transplantation, and these changes have been directly associated with glucocorticoid dose. Bone mineral densities decline rapidly after lung transplantation, and it has been reported that 73% of patients after lung transplantation exhibit reductions in bone mineral density sufficient for the diagnosis of osteoporosis [13]. One-third of lung transplant patients may suffer vertebral fractures. As noted above, patients with chronic lung disease often are exposed to substantial corticosteroid doses before lung transplantation, and their catabolic effects on bone are exaggerated by increases in corticosteroids in the posttransplant period. Reductions in bone mineral density have also been reported in the first year after liver transplantation [15]. Up to one-third of liver transplant patients may experience vertebral fractures. As in other solid organ transplantations, the extent of pretransplant bone disease and the posttransplant immunosuppressive regimen have substantial influence on posttransplant osteoporosis and fractures.

Posttransplant immunosuppressive regimens, especially the use of corticosteroids, appear to play central roles in the development of posttransplantation bone loss and concomitant fractures. Corticosteroids have numerous deleterious effects on skeletal metabolism, resulting in a net loss of bone strength and structure, and contributing to increases in fracture risk. Corticosteroids inhibit the formation of osteoblasts as well as synthetic activities performed by osteoblasts, both of organic matrix and mineralization. Corticosteroids decrease the differentiation of marrow stromal cells into osteoblasts. In a number of animal models of both osteoporosis and avascular necrosis, corticosteroids cause a differentiation of stromal cells away from an osteoblastic and toward an adipocytic lineage. Corticosteroids inhibit the synthesis by osteocytes of type 1 collagen, a major constituent of osteoid. Corticosteroids also induce apoptosis of osteoblasts. All of these effects contribute to a reduction in the number of mature osteocytes and decreased bone formation. Corticosteroids also affect the systemic metabolism of calcium, and exert a downward pressure on calcium homeostasis by decreasing calcium absorption in the gastrointestinal tract and increasing urinary excretion of calcium. The result of these cellular and metabolic changes is a low-turnover osteoporosis and a net loss of bone mineral density, especially within the first year after corticosteroid exposure. Because turnover of trabecular bone is faster than that of cortical bone, the effects of corticosteroid-induced bone suppression are seen initially in trabecular bone, with an increased risk of vertebral fractures. Bone loss appears to be related to corticosteroid dose; investigators differ on the relative importance of mean, peak, and cumulative dose and duration of exposure.

In recent years, other immunosuppressive agents have been introduced that reduce the need for corticosteroids. Prominent among these are the calcineurin inhibitors, cyclosporine and tacrolimus. Immunosuppressants in this class prevent cytokine transcription by T-lymphocytes. However, these agents also have catabolic effects on the skeleton, and may cause substantial reductions in bone mineral density [16,17]. Unlike corticosteroids, these agents can cause high-turnover osteoporosis, and accelerated rates of bone turnover and reductions in bone mineral density are seen within the first year after exposure to these immunosuppressant agents. High-turnover osteoporosis has been seen with these agents in all solid-organ transplantations, including the kidney. When calcineurin inhibitors are used with corticosteroids, high-turnover bone loss may, in fact, predominate over the low-turnover bone loss induced by corticosteroids [18,19]. The incidence of fractures has been concomitantly high in patients treated with calcineurin inhibitors.

The accelerated bone loss and relatively high fracture rates observed in the first year after organ transplantation are undoubtedly multifactorial, reflecting the presence of chronic disease, decreased calcium and vitamin D intake, and relative immobilization. Fractures add substantial morbidity to the posttransplant period. The presence of reduced bone mineral density pretransplantation must be recognized, and rapid bone loss following transplantation should be anticipated. Monitoring and pharmacologic intervention are required to reduce fracture incidence and morbidity.

## Renal osteodystrophy and kidney transplantation

Chronic renal failure is associated with several serious abnormalities in bone metabolism, collectively known as renal osteodystrophy. Renal osteodystrophy refers to the constellation of hyperparathyroidism, osteomalacia, and a combination of the two known as mixed uremic osteodystrophy. Hyperparathyroidism is associated with accelerated bone turnover with a net loss of bone. Osteomalacia is associated with low bone turnover, a failure of osteoid mineralization, and a net loss of bone. Mixed uremic osteodystrophy, as the name implies, consists of decreased bone density with varying contributions of hyperparathyroidism and mineralization failure. In all three forms, patients complain of bone pain and experience an increased incidence of fracture, often with delayed fracture healing. Iliac crest bone biopsy is often helpful in determining the histologic type of renal osteodystrophy. Attention is paid to trabecular morphology, osteoid borders, osteoblast and osteoclast activity, and the mineralization front (with double tetracycline labeling).

Histomorphometric features associated with hyperparathyroidism include osteoclastic bone resorption, marrow fibrosis, trabecular cavitation, and bone loss (Fig. 4). When repair bone is observed, it is primarily of

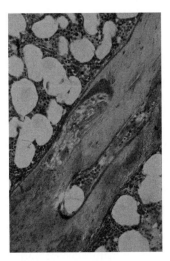

Fig. 4. Iliac crest bone biopsy of hyperparathyroidism. Osteoclastic bone resorption and loss of trabecular structure are histologic hallmarks.

the immature, woven type, and is not well organized along lines of applied force. The net result is a decrease in both cortical and trabecular bone, loss of biomechanical strength, bone pain, and fracture. Mineralization failure, often termed low-turnover osteomalacia or adynamic bone disease, is associated with unmineralized osteoid and an increase in the length and width of osteoid seams on trabeculae (Fig. 5). Bone turnover is low, with an overall

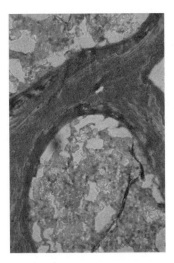

Fig. 5. Iliac crest bone biopsy in osteomalacia. Thick osteoid seams are noted lining the trabecular surfaces. The length of trabecular surface covered with unmineralized osteoid is markedly increased in osteomalacia.

net loss of bone, bone pain, and fractures. Variable amounts of osteomalacia and hyperparathyroidism may coexist in the syndrome of mixed uremic osteodystrophy. Bone biopsies may show one or more of the following characteristics of high turnover bone loss and mineralization failure: (1) decreased trabecular volume, (2) increase in osteoid border length and width, (3) osteoclastic bone resorption, and (4) failure of the mineralization front. As in the other forms of renal osteodystrophy, patients may experience bone pain and fractures.

After kidney transplantation, pretransplantation renal osteodystrophy may not be completely reversed. As in other solid-organ transplantations, rapid bone loss during the first year after kidney transplantation has been observed. Loss of bone mineral density in the first year after kidney transplantation has been reported to be from 5% to 10% [20,21]. In fact, fracture rates after kidney transplantation have been reported to range from 18 to 34 times higher than those of the normal population [3]. Factors contributing to the loss of bone mineral density and concomitant risk of fracture after kidney transplantation include the extent of pretransplantation osteodystrophy, posttransplant immunosuppression, and persistent hyperparathyroidism not corrected by kidney transplantation. Persistent hyperparathyroidism is not uncommon after kidney transplantation and may require treatment intervention. Persistent hyperparathyroidism is associated with high-turnover bone disease, loss of bone mineral density, and fracture. The persistence of osteomalacia or low-turnover bone disease after kidney transplantation may be related to immunosuppressive regimens, primarily corticosteroids. Corticosteroids decrease the number of osteoblasts and reduce the ability of osteoblasts to make and mineralize osteoid. The result is persisting low bone mineral density, bone pain, and fractures.

## Treatment of transplant-associated bone disease

The treatment of decreased bone density in the transplant setting depends upon recognition of existing pretransplantation bone disease and anticipating rapid loss of bone density after transplantation. From the point of view of bone, optimal immunosuppressive regimens have not yet been devised. Treatment falls into two categories: (1) optimizing bone health, and (2) correction of specific metabolic deficits. Bone health can be optimized by maintaining a daily calcium intake of 1200 to 1500 mg and a vitamin D intake of 400 to 800 IU. Calcium and vitamin D supplementation is particularly useful in patients with osteomalacia and attendant mineralization failure. Unmineralized osteoid usually mineralizes once calcium and vitamin D intake is optimized. Weight-bearing exercise, typically in the form of walking, should be encouraged, even with the accompanying chronic disease pretransplantation and certainly posttransplantation. Many specific defects associated with solid organ transplantations are, in fact, corrected by the transplant. In particular, successful transplantation facilitates weight-bearing exercise programs. Patients should stop smoking and moderate their use of caffeine. Several pharmacologic agents are available to increase bone density. Calcitonin is an antiresorptive agent that reduces bone loss and is particularly helpful in reducing bone pain. Recombinant parathyroid hormone fragments such as teriparatide—rhPTH(1–34)—may be particularly useful in patients with low bone turnover states. Bisphosphonates are now widely used to treat bone loss after transplantation.

Renal osteodystrophy consists of hyperparathyroidism and osteomalacia in varying combinations, resulting in a spectrum of bone turnover states from high to low. Renal osteodystrophy can be complicated by the superimposition of catabolic effects on bone by immunosuppression. The treatment of renal osteodystrophy should ideally begin before transplantation and continue afterward [22–24]. Hyperphosphatemia should be corrected, and calcium and vitamin D intake should be optimized. Bisphosphonates can be used to increase bone density, and are the most effective agents for restoring bone mass after transplantation. Persistent mild hyperparathyroidism can often be corrected with calcium and vitamin D; serum vitamin D levels should be 20 to 40 ng/mL. Persistent severe hyperparathyroidism associated with hypercalcemia is amenable to treatment by parathyroidectomy. Mineralization defects, however, should be corrected first if possible, because correction after parathyroidectomy may be difficult.

The correction of reduced bone density after transplantation is complicated by immunosuppressive regimens, particularly corticosteroids. Corticosteroids suppress bone formation rates, increase bone resorption, decrease gastrointestinal absorption of calcium, and induce hypercalciuria in a dose-dependent manner. Wherever feasible, the dose and duration of corticosteroid exposure should be minimized. Bisphosphonates, together with optimized calcium and vitamin D intake, appear to be useful for the management of corticosteroid-associated bone loss. Studies with etidronate, alendronate, and risedronate have shown that all these agents reduce bone resorption and increase bone density. Intravenous pamidronate is also useful, and may be particularly so in individuals with gastrointestinal intolerance to oral bisphosphonates. Intermittent teriparatide may also be useful in increasing bone mass. The effects of these agents on reduction of fracture risk, however, have not been well studied.

## Organ transplantation and avascular necrosis

Although avascular necrosis (AVN) may affect several joints, including the knee, shoulder, and ankle, AVN of the femoral head is the most common and severe form of the disease and has the most relevance to a discussion of organ transplant complications. AVN of the femoral head refers to the death of osteocytes, with subsequent structural changes leading to femoral head collapse and secondary hip joint osteoarthritis [25]. AVN of the femoral head is now recognized to be a relatively common disorder, accounting for 5% to 10% of total hip replacements done in the United States [26,27]. It occurs in various series in 5% to 25% of patients taking corticosteroids [26]. The male-to-female ratio is approximately 4:1, and the mean age of onset is in the fifth decade. The presentation of symptoms may be asynchronous, but because bilaterality occurs regardless of the temporal appearance of symptoms, a high index of suspicion must be maintained for disease bilaterality. Pain is the usual presenting symptom, and can be very intense and sudden in onset, as in an infarct, or it can be insidious and chronic. It is most often reported in the groin, but radiating pain to the anterior or anteromedial thigh is common. Buttock pain may be reported. On physical examination, a corresponding decrease in range of motion, particularly flexion and internal rotation, is observed. Except in the case of certain specific etiologies (e.g., hemoglobinopathies), laboratory studies are normal.

The most widely used radiographic staging system for AVN is the Ficat classification [28]. Stage 0 denotes an asymptomatic, preradiographic (radiographically normal) hip with positive diagnostic imaging studies, such as MRI or technetium bone scan. Stage I denotes a symptomatic hip with normal radiographs and positive diagnostic imaging studies. Stage II hips exhibit alterations in trabecular pattern of mottled sclerosis and lucency without subchondral fracture or change in femoral head contour. Stage III consists of hips in which a subchondral fracture (crescent sign) or subchondral collapse occurs with a loss of sphericity and change in contour of the femoral head. Stage IV is synonymous with secondary osteoarthritis. MRI is the standard for functional imaging; the T1 images show low-intensity signal, and the T2 images exhibit signals of alternating high and low intensity, the so-called double-line sign (Fig. 6).

## Etiology and progression of avascular necrosis

Several etiologies of nontraumatic AVN have been proposed, including dysbarism (changes in ambient pressure), alcohol, hemoglobinopathies, and corticosteroids. AVN associated with corticosteroid administration is of most interest in the clinical setting of organ transplantation. Steroid-associated AVN accounts for 10% to 30% of AVN cases, depending on the center reporting. A meta-analysis of 22 studies of steroid-associated AVN found no correlation between the underlying associated disease and the AVN, although it did determine a 4.6-fold increase in AVN occurrence for every 10 mg/d increase in oral corticosteroid intake [29]. Corticosteroids have long been implicated as an etiologic association in AVN because AVN is associated with corticosteroid intake in a number of diverse conditions including lupus, rheumatoid arthritis, asthma, organ transplantation, and Cushing's disease. Although it is not certain that the use of corticosteroids presents equal risks in various conditions, clinical attention has been focused on identifying a threshold dose of corticosteroids in determining risk for

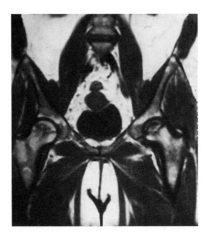

Fig. 6. MRI of the hip in avascular necrosis. These coronal sections demonstrate alternating areas of high and low signal intensity, pathognomic of avascular necrosis. (*From* Aaron RK, Gray RRL. Osteonecrosis: etiology, natural history, pathophysiology, and diagnosis. In: Callaghan JJ, Rosenberg AJ, Rubash HE, editors. The adult hip. 2nd edition. Philadelphia (PA): Lippincott Williams & Wilkins, 2006.)

AVN. Dose can be expressed as mean daily, peak, or cumulative (total) dose, and duration of exposure. Most studies have suggested an association of AVN with mean daily or peak dose and have reported that high doses, even for short duration, present more significant risks than cumulative dose or duration of therapy. One study of 161 patients with inflammatory bowel disease treated with corticosteroids reported an AVN incidence of 4.3%. The mean daily prednisone dose was 26 mg/d (range = 12 to 34 mg/d), the mean duration of treatment was 42 weeks (range = 20 to 84 weeks), and the mean cumulative prednisone dose was 7000 mg (range = 1800 to 13,500 mg) [30]. In a series of 110 patients with steroid-associated AVN with various diseases, the cumulative prednisone dose was 42 g [31]. In a series of patients with steroid-associated AVN in lupus, the mean daily dose was greater than 20 mg/d, and the mean cumulative prednisone dose was 45 g with a mean duration of treatment of 260 weeks [32]. In heart transplant patients, no association between the development of AVN and cumulative prednisone dose was found, but there was an association between AVN and the peak dose of methylprednisolone [33]. The situation may be more complicated in renal transplant patients because of the presence of renal osteodystrophy, but it is probable that AVN in this patient population is largely related to the mean daily steroid dose [34]. Most patients with AVN in these and other studies received mean daily doses of greater than 20 mg/d, and that dose is generally regarded as presenting a significant risk for AVN [29,30,32,35].

Some studies have suggested that AVN associated with corticosteroid intake, particularly in organ transplant patients, is characterized by a less complete repair process, with suppressed bone production [27,36]. Iliac crest bone biopsies of patients with AVN from various etiologies including transplantation demonstrate a histologic profile consistent with osteoporosis, including a reduction in trabecular bone volume and osteoid seam width, a decrease in osteoblastic appositional rate and bone formation rate, and an increase in total resorptive surface [37]. No histopathologic differences based on presumed etiology were observed.

A unifying concept of the pathogenesis of AVN emphasizes the central role of vascular occlusion and ischemia leading to osteocyte necrosis [38]. Decreased femoral head blood flow can occur through three mechanisms: vascular interruption (fractures or dislocation), extravascular compression (by lipocyte hypertrophy and marrow fat deposition), and thrombotic occlusion (by intravascular thrombi or embolic fat). A number of studies have demonstrated that, particularly after corticosteroid administration, lipids deposit in the marrow extravascular space and within osteocytes and can create an elevation of intraosseous extravascular pressure [39]. Hypertrophy and proliferation of adipocytes have been shown in both patients and experimental animals with AVN associated with corticosteroid administration [40–42]. Adipocyte hypertrophy and hyperplasia and intraosseous, extravascular lipid deposition are thought to result in intraosseous hypertension and diminished blood flow [39]. Corticosteroid administration may also decrease the number of osteoprogenitor cells by shifting precursors from an osteocytic to an adipocytic pathway. Studies using a cloned mouse bone marrow progenitor cell line have indicated that adipocytes and osteocytes share a common progenitor cell, but in corticosteroid- or alcohol-induced adipogenesis, cells shunt from the osteocytic to the adipocytic lineage [43]. This may contribute to the reduced ability of osteocytes to effect bone repair.

Despite a variety of pathogenic mechanisms, all forms of AVN eventually converge to a more or less consistent histopathology. Although osteocyte necrosis occurs after 2 to 3 hours of anoxia, 24 to 72 hours are necessary for the appearance of histologic signs of osteocyte death [36,44–46]. The earliest findings of AVN on light microscopy are hematopoietic marrow, adipocyte necrosis, and interstitial edema [46,47]. Osteocyte necrosis is reflected by pyknosis of nuclei and subsequently by empty osteocyte lacunae (Fig. 7). The necrotic area is surrounded by a zone of reactive hyperemia [48]. Capillary neogenesis and revascularization occur to a degree peripheral to the necrotic zone [25,49]. With the entry of blood vessels into the zone of necrosis, a repair process begins consisting of coupled bone resorption and production that produces the radiographic appearance of sclerosis and lucency [36,49–52]. In the cancellous bone, proliferation of capillaries is observed, and new living bone is laminated onto dead trabeculae with partial resorption of the dead bone (Fig. 8) [38]. In the subchondral area, bone formation occurs at a slower rate than does resorption, resulting in the net loss of bone and structural integrity, subchondral fracture, and collapse. The radiographic appearance of lucency represents zones of bone

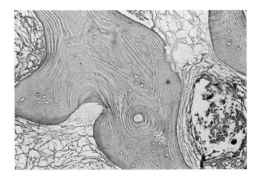

Fig. 7. Histopathology of avascular necrosis. Histologic section of the subchondral bone exhibiting dead trabeculae with empty osteocyte lacunae and hemorrhagic marrow with necrosis.

resorption; areas of sclerosis are composed of both dead and living reparative bone laminated on dead trabeculae (Fig. 9). Resorption of bone may also cause fractures either in a subchondral location or deep in the femoral head leading to segmental collapse. It is not the osteocyte necrosis per se but rather the repair process and the imbalance between bone resorption and formation that leads to the loss of structural integrity of the femoral head.

Clinical progression occurs equally in Ficat grades I, II, and III. By the 36-month follow-up, 54% of stage I, 66% of stage II, and 73% of stage III hips require hip replacement surgery. The mean times to clinical failure are 27 months for stage I, 24 months for stage II, and 21 months for stage III hips. Radiographic progression also occurs equally in all three Ficat grades; by the 36-month follow-up, 94% of stage I, 83% of stage II, and 92% of stage III hips had progressed radiographically. In one study, 57 hips (71%) progressed clinically and 91% of hips progressed radiographically [53]. It is possible that the radiographic progression of Ficat stage I

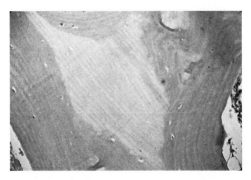

Fig. 8. Histologic section demonstrating lamination of living bone upon a section of dead trabeculae. Note the presence of osteocytes in the lacunae of living bone. (*From* Aaron RK, Gray RRL. Osteonecrosis: etiology, natural history, pathophysiology, and diagnosis. In: Callaghan JJ, Rosenberg AJ, Rubash HE, editors. The adult hip. 2nd edition. Philadelphia (PA): Lippincott Williams & Wilkins, 2006.)

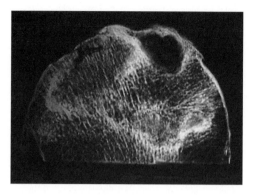

Fig. 9. Specimen radiograph showing details of sclerotic and lucent zones. The sclerotic zones are composed of living bone laminated on dead trabeculae. Subchondral fracture is evident with 1 mm of collapse. (*From* Aaron RK, Gray RRL. Osteonecrosis: etiology, natural history, pathophysiology, and diagnosis. In: Callaghan JJ, Rosenberg AJ, Rubash HE, editors. The adult hip. 2nd edition. Philadelphia (PA): Lippincott Williams & Wilkins, 2006.)

and II lesions, respectively, have entirely different prognostic significance. Radiographic progression of Ficat stage I lesions implies the appearance of a previously preradiographic lesion, whereas progression of Ficat stage II lesions indicates structural failure (i.e., subchondral fracture). However, the correlation of radiographic and clinical progression and the similar rates of clinical progression in both groups suggest that radiographic progression is clinically significant in Ficat I hips. Within the first 2 years of follow-up, Ficat stage II and III hips exhibited more rapid collapse compared with Ficat stage I hips, but at the 36-month follow-up, all three groups exhibited similar rates of progression, with 64% to 72% of hips exhibiting collapse in the three groups. The mean time to collapse was 22 months for Ficat stage I hips, 16 months for Ficat stage II hips, and 20 months for Ficat stage III hips.

AVN is a disabling and progressive condition, and leads to femoral head collapse usually requiring total hip replacement. Because hip-preserving therapies are most effective in the earliest stages of AVN before subchondral fracture, the key to successful treatment lies in identifying at-risk populations and quantifying their risk in terms of clinical and pathophysiologic characteristics so that early diagnosis can be made before femoral head collapse [38].

*Treatment of avascular necrosis associated with organ transplantation*

AVN is a progressive condition that, if untreated, results in joint collapse, incongruity, and secondary osteoarthritis. Pain associated with end-stage AVN usually requires joint replacement. Because of chronic disease, immunosuppression, and diminished bone density, the complications of total joint replacement are increased in the transplant population. AVN occurs with greatest frequency in the hip, followed by the knee, shoulder, and ankle.

Most studies done on the treatment of AVN have been done on the hip, and the following discussion centers on the femoral head, although it can be extrapolated, with cautions, to other joints.

The ability to preserve the femoral head depends upon the stage at which AVN is detected. From the point of view of joint preservation, staging can be divided into those joints without structural failure (fracture or collapse), in which preservation is possible, and those with failure, in which preservation is not usually accomplished. Hip preservation has been attempted with structural grafts, which may be vascularized or nonvascularized, or osteoinductive grafting of cancellous autograft. Autologous fibular grafting with microvascular anastomoses has been successful [54]. Recently, emphasis has been placed on resorption of subchondral trabeculae as the key pathophysiologic event leading to femoral head collapse [55]. This observation has provided a rationale for the use of antiresorptive therapy with bisphosphonates or electric fields to alter the balance of bone remodeling from resorption to formation. Early data has indicated that progression to fracture and collapse can be prevented by antiresorptive therapy.

Methods for surgical treatment of avascular necrosis of the femoral head have recently been treated in several reviews. These methods include core decompression with or without biologic augmentation, nonvascularized bone grafts, vascularized fibular grafting, intertrochanteric osteotomy, and total hip replacement [54–59].

The surgical procedure of core decompression creates a core track from the lateral femoral cortex to the osteonecrotic lesion. A variety of strategies have been devised to enhance osteogenesis in the core track, including autogenous cancellous graft, osteoinductive substances, and vascularized fibular grafting. The results of core decompression reveal considerable variability in clinical and radiographic outcomes with satisfactory results limited largely to precollapse lesions. In general, 80% to 90% of precollapse (Stage I) hips, 60% to 65% of radiographically apparent precollapse hips (Stage II), and 30% to 45% of postcollapse hips have experienced satisfactory clinical or radiographic outcomes. The biomechanical effects of core decompression have been studied with regard both to core placement and depth of penetration into the osteonecrotic lesions, and it has been demonstrated that an inappropriately placed core track can increase stresses in the subchondral bone and increase the risk of local collapse. Results in postcollapse hips are not substantially different from those receiving nonoperative treatment, and core decompression is now rarely recommended for lesions with subchondral fracture with or without collapse. Core decompression has been combined with osteoinductive grafting with autogenous graft or demineralized bone matrix, and, while the results in small series have been encouraging, it has been difficult to demonstrate clear superiority of these techniques over core decompression alone. Supplementary antiresorptive therapy with either bisphosphonates or electrical stimulation shows some benefit in precollapse hips in small series.

Total hip replacement has been used in the treatment of avascular necrosis of the femoral head for failures of hip-preserving therapy or in patients who present with postcollapse lesions with or without joint involvement. Most total hip replacements for avascular necrosis are performed with uncemented femoral and acetabular components. However, in patients with substantial bone loss due to corticosteroid-induced or other metabolic bone circumstances including renal osteodystrophy, cemented femoral components may be used. Chronic illnesses, including decreased bone density, have an adverse outcome on the results of total hip replacement. Patients with idiopathic avascular necrosis experience satisfactory clinical results in approximately 92% of cases. By contrast, similarly good clinical results were observed in only 78% of renal transplant patients with avascular necrosis and in 63% of patients with steroid-induced avascular necrosis associated with systemic lupus erythematosus [60]. Other studies have demonstrated high failure rate of total hip replacement in patients with chronic dialysis, including an infection rate of 19% and a revision rate of 31% of cemented hips in patients with renal transplantation. By contrast, good results have been reported from uncemented total hip replacements in kidney transplant patients [61–63]. The general consensus is that patients with kidney transplantation—and, presumably, underlying renal osteodystrophy and contribution of corticosteroid-induced osteoporosis—still do reasonably well after total hip replacement, although failure rates are somewhat higher than those of patients with idiopathic avascular necrosis or osteoarthritis. Uncemented hip replacements are generally preferable in patients under 50 years of age, whereas cemented hip replacements may be useful in patients with significant bone loss.

## References

[1] Black DM, Steinbuch M, Palermo L, et al. An assessment tool for predicting fracture risk in postmenopausal women. Osteoporos Int 2001;12(7):519–28.

[2] Kanis JA, Johnell O, Oden A, et al. Ten-year probabilities of osteoporotic fractures according to BMD and diagnostic thresholds. Osteoporos Int 2001;12(12):989–95.

[3] Ramsey-Goldman R, Dunn JE, Dunlop DD, et al. Increased risk of fracture in patients receiving solid organ transplants. J Bone Miner Res 1999;14(3):456–63.

[4] Van Cleemput J, Daenen W, Nijs J, et al. Timing and quantification of bone loss in cardiac transplant recipients. Transpl Int 1995;8(3):196–200.

[5] Ippoliti G, Pellegrini C, Campana C, et al. Clodronate treatment of established bone loss in cardiac recipients: a randomized study. Transplantation 2003;75(3):330–4.

[6] Leidig-Bruckner G, Hosch S, Dodidou P, et al. Frequency and predictors of osteoporotic fractures after cardiac or liver transplantation: a follow-up study. Lancet 2001;357(9253): 342–7.

[7] Shane E, Papadopoulos A, Staron RB, et al. Bone loss and fracture after lung transplantation. Transplantation 1999;68(2):220–7.

[8] Aris RM, Lester GE, Renner JB, et al. Efficacy of pamidronate for osteoporosis in patients with cystic fibrosis following lung transplantation. Am J Respir Crit Care Med 2000; 162(3 Pt 1):941–6.

[9] Porayko MD, Wiesner RH, Hay JE, et al. Bone disease in liver transplant recipients: incidence, timing, and risk factors. Transplant Proc 1991;23(1 Pt 2):1462–5.

[10] Heidrich FE, Stergachis A, Gross KM. Diuretic drug use and the risk for hip fracture. Ann Intern Med 1991;115(1):1–6.

[11] Caraballo PJ, Heit JA, Atkinson EJ, et al. Long-term use of oral anticoagulants and the risk of fracture. Arch Intern Med 1999;159(15):1750–6.

[12] Shane E, Silverberg SJ, Donovan D, et al. Osteoporosis in lung transplantation candidates with end-stage pulmonary disease. Am J Med 1996;101(3):262–9.

[13] Aris RM, Neuringer IP, Weiner MA, et al. Severe osteoporosis before and after lung transplantation. Chest 1996;109(5):1176–83.

[14] Shane R, Rivas M, Staron RB, et al. Fracture after cardiac transplantation: a prospective longitudinal study. J Clin Endocrinol Metab 1996;81(5):1740–6.

[15] Monegal A, Navasa M, Guañabens N, et al. Bone disease after liver transplantation: a long-term prospective study of bone mass changes, hormonal disorders, and histomorphometric characteristics. Osteoporos Int 2001;12(6):484–92.

[16] Movsowitz C, Epstein S, Fallon M, et al. Cyclosporin-A in vivo produces severe osteopenia in the rat: effect of dose and duration of administration. Endocrinology 1988;123(5):2571–7.

[17] Movsowitz C, Epstein S, Ismail F, et al. Cyclosporin-A in the oophorectomized rat: unexpected severe bone resorption. J Bone Miner Res 1989;4(3):393–8.

[18] Thiebaud D, Krieg MA, Gillard-Berguer D, et al. Cyclosporine induces high bone turnover and may contribute to bone loss after heart transplantation. Eur J Clin Invest 1996;26(7):549–55.

[19] Aubia J, Masramon J, Serrano S, et al. Bone histology in renal transplant patients receiving cyclosporine. Lancet 1988;1:1048–9.

[20] Almond MK, Kwan JT, Evans K, et al. Loss of regional bone mineral density in the first 12 months following renal transplantation. Nephron 1994;66(1):52–7.

[21] Dalen N, Alvestrand A. Bone mineral content in chronic renal failure and after renal transplantation. Clin Nephrol 1973;1(6):338–46.

[22] Eknoyan G, Levin A, Levin NW. Bone metabolism and disease in chronic kidney disease. Am J Kidney Dis 2003;42(Suppl 3):S1–201.

[23] Elder G. Pathophysiology and recent advances in the management of renal osteodystrophy. J Bone Miner Res 2002;17(12):2094–105.

[24] Cunningham J, Sprague SM, Cannata-Andia J, et al. Osteoporosis in chronic kidney disease. Am J Kidney Dis 2004;43(3):566–71.

[25] Jones JP Jr. Etiology and pathogenesis of osteonecrosis. Semin Arthroplasty 1991;2:160–8.

[26] Mankin HJ. Nontraumatic necrosis of bone (osteonecrosis). N Engl J Med 1992;326(22):1473–9.

[27] Zizic TM, Hungerford DS. Avascular necrosis of bone. In: Kelly WN, Harris ED, Ruddy S, Sledge CB, editors. Textbook of rheumatology. Philadelphia (PA): WB Saunders; 1985. p. 1689–710.

[28] Ficat RP. Idiopathic bone necrosis of the femoral head: early diagnosis and treatment. J Bone Joint Surg 1985;67B(1):3–9.

[29] Felson T, Anderson J. A cross-study evaluation of association between steroid dose and bolus steroids and avascular necrosis of bone. Lancet 1987;1(8538):902–6.

[30] Vakil N, Sparberg M. Steroid-related osteonecrosis in inflammatory bowel disease. Gastroenterology 1989;96(1):62–7.

[31] Cruess RL. Steroid-induced osteonecrosis. J R Coll Surg Edinb 1981;26(2):69–77.

[32] Zizic TM, Marcoux C, Hungerford DS, et al. Corticosteroid therapy associated with ischemic necrosis of bone in systemic lupus erythematosus. Am J Med 1985;79(5):596–603.

[33] Bradbury G, Benjamin J, Thompson J, et al. Avascular necrosis of bone after cardiac transplantation. J Bone Joint Surg 1994;76A(9):1385–8.

[34] Landmann J, Renner N, Gachter A, et al. Cyclosporin A and osteonecrosis of the femoral head. J Bone Joint Surg 1987;69A(8):1226–8.

[35] Fisher DE, Bickel WH. Corticosteroid-induced avascular necrosis: a clinical study of seventy-seven patients. J Bone Joint Surg 1971;53A(5):859–73.

[36] Kenzora JE, Glimcher MJ. Osteonecrosis. In: Kelley WN, Harris ED, Russy S, Sledge CB, editors. Textbook of rheumatology. Philadelphia (PA): WB Saunders; 1981. p. 1755–82.

[37] Arlot M, Bonjean M, Chavassieux P, et al. Bone histology in adults with aseptic necrosis. J Bone Joint Surg 1983;65A(9):1319–27.

[38] Aaron RK, Gray RRL. Osteonecrosis: etiology, natural history, pathophysiology, and diagnosis. In: Callaghan JJ, Rosenberg AG, Rubash HE, editors. The adult hip. 2nd edition. Philadelphia (PA): Lippincott Williams & Wilkins; in press.

[39] Wang GJ, Cui Q, Balian G. The pathogenesis and prevention of steroid-induced osteonecrosis. Clin Orthop Rel Res 2000;370:295–310.

[40] Kawai K, Tamaki A, Hirohata K. Steroid-induced accumulation of lipid in the osteocytes of the rabbit femoral head: a histochemical and electron microscopic study. J Bone Joint Surg 1985;67A(5):755–63.

[41] Wang GJ, Lennox DW, Reger SI, et al. Cortisone-induced intrafemoral head pressure change and its response to a drilling decompression method. Clin Orthop 1981;159:274–8.

[42] Wang GJ, Sweet D, Reger SI, et al. Fat cell changes as a mechanism of avascular necrosis of the femoral head in cortisone-treated rabbits. J Bone Joint Surg 1977;59A(6):729–35.

[43] Wang Y, Li Y, Mao K, et al. Alcohol-induced adipogenesis in bone and marrow: a possible mechanism for osteonecrosis. Clin Orthop Rel Res 2003;410:213–24.

[44] Bauer TW, Stulberg BN. The histology of osteonecrosis and its distinction from histologic artifacts. In: Schoutens A, Arlet J, Gardeniers JWM, et al, editors. Bone circulation and vascularization in normal and pathological conditions. New York: Plenum Press; 1993. p. 283–92.

[45] James J, Steijn-Myagkaya GL. Death of osteocytes: electron microscopy after in vitro ischaemia. J Bone Joint Surg 1986;68B(4):620–4.

[46] Jones JP Jr. Osteonecrosis. In: McCarty DJ, editor. Arthritis and allied conditions. Philadelphia (PA): Lea & Febiger; 1985. p. 1356–73.

[47] Saito S, Inoue A, Ono K. Intramedullary hemorrhage as a possible cause of avascular necrosis of the femoral head. J Bone Joint Surg 1987;69B(3):346–51.

[48] Sissons HA, Nuovo MA, Steiner GC. Pathology of osteonecrosis of the femoral head. Skeletal Radiol 1992;21(4):229–38.

[49] Glimcher MJ, Kenzora JE. The biology of osteonecrosis of the human femoral head and its clinical implications: I. Tissue biology. Clin Orthop 1979;138:284–309.

[50] Glimcher MJ, Kenzora JE. The biology of osteonecrosis of the human femoral head and its clinical implications. II. The pathological changes in the femoral head as an organ and in the hip joint. Clin Orthop 1979;139:283–312.

[51] Glimcher MJ, Kenzora JE. The biology of osteonecrosis of the human femoral head and its clinical implications. III. Discussion of the etiology and genesis of the pathological sequelae; comments on treatment. Clin Orthop 1979;140:273–312.

[52] Catto M. A histological study of avascular necrosis of the femoral head after transcervical fracture. J Bone Joint Surg 1965;47B(4):749–53.

[53] Aaron RK, Stulberg BN, Lennox DW. Clinical and radiographic outcomes in untreated symptomatic osteonecrosis of the femoral head. Tech Orthop 2001;16(1):1–5.

[54] Katz MA, Urbaniak JR. Free vascularized fibular grafting of the femoral head for the treatment of osteonecrosis. Tech Orthop 2001;16(1):44–60.

[55] Brown TD. Biomechanical aspects of subchondral fracture, core decompression, and bone grafting in femoral head osteonecrosis. Tech Orthop 2001;16(1):16–23.

[56] Stulberg BN. Optimizing the outcome of core decompression. Tech Orthop 2001;16(1):24–31.

[57] Ciombor DM, Aaron RK. Biologically augmented core decompression for the treatment of osteonecrosis of the femoral head. Tech Orthop 2001;16(1):32–8.

[58] Etienne G, Mont MA, Khanuja HS, et al. Nonvascularized bone grafts for osteonecrosis of the femoral head: current concepts and techniques. Tech Orthop 2001;16(1):39–43.

[59] Sanchez A, Khatod M, Santore R. The role of intertrochanteric osteotomy in the treatment of osteonecrosis. Tech Orthop 2001;16(1):61–5.

[60] Brinker MR, Rosenberg AG, Kull L, et al. Primary total hip arthroplasty using noncemented porous-coated femoral components in patients with osteonecrosis of the femoral head. J Arthroplasty 1994;9(5):457–68.

[61] Alpert B, Waddell JP, Morton J, et al. Cementless total hip arthroplasty in renal transplant patients. Clin Orthop 1992;284:164–9.

[62] Lieberman JR, Fuchs MD, Haas SB, et al. Hip arthroplasty in patients with chronic renal failure. J Arthroplasty 1995;10(2):191–5.

[63] Murzic WJ, McCollum DE. Hip arthroplasty for osteonecrosis after renal transplantation. Clin Orthop 1994;299:212–9.

SURGICAL
CLINICS OF
NORTH AMERICA

Surg Clin N Am 86 (2006) 1257–1276

# Skin Cancer After Transplantation: A Guide for the General Surgeon

Kevan G. Lewis, MD, MS[a], Nathaniel Jellinek, MD[a],
Leslie Robinson-Bostom, MD[a,b,*]

[a]*Department of Dermatology, Brown Medical School/Rhode Island Hospital,
593 Eddy Street, APC-10, Providence, RI 02903, USA*
[b]*Department of Pathology, Brown Medical School/Rhode Island Hospital-APC 10,
593 Eddy Street, Providence, RI 02903, USA*

The success of organ transplantation has been accompanied by serious concerns regarding the incidence and management of potentially catastrophic cutaneous carcinogenesis in transplant recipients. Delivery of the highest quality of care requires a concerted effort toward collaboration between multiple surgical and medical specialties. The purpose of this review is to provide the general surgeon with a practical, user-friendly guide to the important components of comprehensive dermatologic care for organ transplant recipients (OTRs) with references to more detailed sources of information.

The following learning objectives have been established for the reader:

- What is the scope of the problem in this patient population?
- What is the biology of cutaneous oncogenesis?
- How is iatrogenic immunosuppression related to cutaneous carcinogenesis?
- What are the risk factors for skin cancer in OTRs?
- How does history of skin cancer affect the pre-transplant evaluation of potential candidates for organ transplantation?
- What measures can be taken to prevent skin cancer in the post-transplant period?
- What is the optimal management of skin cancer in OTRs?
- When is a reduction of immunosuppression indicated because of the development of cutaneous malignancy?

* Corresponding author.
*E-mail address:* LRobinson_Bostom@lifespan.org (L. Robinson-Bostom).

0039-6109/06/$ - see front matter © 2006 Elsevier Inc. All rights reserved.
doi:10.1016/j.suc.2006.06.007

- What is the role of systemic retinoid chemoprevention in the management of OTRs who develop skin cancer, and what are the side effects of acitretin?
- How frequently should OTRs be followed by a dermatologist because of the risk of skin cancer?
- How does the implementation of multidisciplinary collaboration help to ensure that OTRs receive the highest quality care?
- How should the emphasis on skin cancer prevention, detection, and treatment evolve during the post-transplant period?

## Background and scope of problem

The burden of skin disease among OTRs is substantial, and it poses an increasing public health concern as the longevity of grafts improves and the number of transplantation surgeries increases each year. Dermatologic complications associated with immunosuppressive therapy have also been shown to adversely affect quality of life among affected individuals [1]. Cutaneous malignancies, in particular, have become a widely recognized problem, and in selected individuals they force a choice between an increased risk of allograft rejection and mortality from metastatic cancer. Skin cancer in the post-transplant period is a virtual certainty for many OTRs, and it is by far the most common malignancy among OTRs [2,3].

More than one million cases of cutaneous malignancy are diagnosed annually in the United States. One nationwide population-based study demonstrated that roughly 1% of all non-melanoma skin cancers occurred in OTRs [4]. The epidemiology of skin cancer in OTRs differs from that of the general population in several important ways: younger patients are at increased risk compared with an age-matched reference group in the general population, beginning as soon as 2 to 5 years after transplantation [4,5]. One study showed that among OTRs with a history of skin cancer before transplantation, more than three quarters (76%) developed additional skin tumors (17 tumors on average) in the post-transplant period [6]. OTRs are also more likely to develop multiple tumors than the general population [5]. The increased risk of skin cancer in the post-transplant period has been shown to be greatest among heart recipients, intermediate among kidney recipients, and lowest (but nevertheless significant) among liver recipients [7–10].

Recent population-based studies reporting the epidemiologic trends of skin cancer have helped to define patterns unique to OTRs and differentiated them from the general population. In contrast to the general population, squamous cell carcinoma (SCC) predominates in OTRs. Whereas the incidence rate ratio of BCC to SCC in the general population typically ranges from 2–4:1 [11,12], the ratio is reversed for OTRs, in whom the rate of SCC generally exceeds that of BCC by a factor of 2 to 3 [4,13–16].

As in the non-immunosuppressed population, the risk of skin cancer increases with age. A biphasic increase in incidence related to age at the time of transplantation was noted in one study [4]. Among older OTRs ($\geq 50$ years) a significant increase in skin cancer risk was observed early in the post-transplant period, peaking in the sixth post-transplant year and declining over time. By contrast, younger OTRs ($< 50$ years) demonstrated little increased risk in the early years, but a significant increase peaking 10 to 12 years post-transplant was observed. A decade after transplantation, the absolute risk for both age groups was remarkably similar. Relative risk (to an age-matched reference group in the general population) was increased in both groups. The relative risk of younger OTRs exceeded 200 times the reference group, much higher than that of older OTRs, owing to the sharp age-related increase in the rate of skin cancer in the general non-immunosuppressed population [4].

These findings suggest that the rapid development of skin cancer in older individuals following the induction of immunosuppression might be attributable to the proliferation of a large number of previously immunosubjugated malignant clones that have accumulated over decades [4]. In addition, the increase in relative risk among younger OTRs suggests that the rate of malignant transformation is likely 200 times greater than the observed incidence of skin cancer owing to the capacity of the immunocompetent host to detect and eliminate clonal proliferation [4].

Significant increases in multiple histologic subtypes of skin cancer have been noted in OTRs, including SCC (65-fold) [7], basal cell carcinoma (BCC; 10-fold), melanoma (3–6.6-fold) [4,7,17,18], Kaposi's sarcoma (KS; 84–97-fold) [4,7], and Merkel cell carcinoma (MCC; not quantified) [19]. Skin cancer in OTRs also tends to be more aggressive and has greater potential to metastasize and threaten life [16,20]. The concern for severe morbidity associated with cutaneous malignancy was illustrated by a series of patients who developed more than 10 distinct primary nonmelanoma skin cancers (NMSCs) in a single year [21]. The widespread disease observed in this subset of patients has been termed "catastrophic carcinomatosis" and occurs more commonly in patients with precursor lesions affecting large anatomical areas such as the arms and legs, a distribution referred to as a "field effect" (Fig. 1). Occurrence of in-transit, regional, and distant metastasis is also more frequent in OTRs who have SCC [21]; 3-year survival in the latter group has been estimated at 56% [20]. Mortality caused by skin cancer among OTRs has been estimated at 5%, of which two-thirds has been attributed to SCC [22]. By contrast, mortality from NMSC in the general population has been estimated at less than one death per 100,000 individuals [23]. Malignancies arising primarily from other organ systems are also increased in the post-transplantation period, including esophagus (relative risk [RR] 4.7), liver (RR 4.8), cervix (RR 6.6), bladder (RR 5.1), and thyroid gland (RR 4.5) [24]. Of note, smaller increases in the risk of breast (RR 1.3) and colon (RR 1.9) cancers were noted in transplant recipients; however,

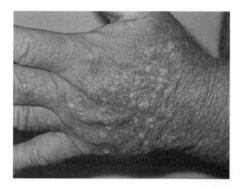

Fig. 1. Dorsal hand showing the characteristic diffuse keratotic papules referred to as the field effect.

27% of deaths occurring at least 4 years after transplantation were caused by skin cancer. This finding suggests that following the post-operative period and stabilization of the immunosuppressant regimen, increased emphasis should be placed on diagnosis and treatment of skin cancer in an effort to reduce mortality from this disease [16].

## Biology of oncogenesis

The pathogenesis of cutaneous malignancy among OTRs, as in the general population, is largely attributable to exposure to excessive UV light [25]. Tumor initiation in keratinocytes is mediated through a series of mutagenic actions on DNA. UV radiation (UVR)-related tumor promotion occurs by way of damage to tumor suppressor genes including p53 and aberrant expression of a host of chemokines, growth factors, pro-inflammatory mediators, and DNA repair enzymes [26,27]. The known carcinogenic and immunosuppressive effects of UV radiation are caused predominantly by exposure to UVB radiation (290–320 nm), the strongest risk factor for skin cancer in the general population. The risk of SCC in azathioprine-treated patients might be related similarly to prior exposure to cutaneous carcinogens including UVB radiation. Exposure to low levels of UVA radiation (320-400 nm) has also been shown to be carcinogenic in the setting of immunosuppression. Azathioprine is converted normally to the active metabolite 6-thioguanine, which is incorporated into the DNA of replicating cells including epidermal keratinocytes; however, exposure to UVA causes 6-thioguanine to be converted to guanine-6-sulfonate ($G-6-SO_3$), reactive oxygen species that induces oxidative stress in the cell and is directly carcinogenic [28]. A sudden increase in reactive oxygen species causes oxidative stress, which (along with $G-6-SO_3$) produces DNA mutations [26,27].

In addition, DNA from the human papillomavirus (HPV) has been isolated in SCC arising in OTRs. The histopathologic architecture of malignant lesions often supports the coexistence of HPV infection. HPV types 1, 2, 5, 16, and 18 have been isolated from warts, actinic keratoses, and SCC arising in kidney transplant recipients [29]. A superfamily of HPV types that were described in association with viral warts and SCC in patients who had the inherited condition epidermodysplasia verruciformis (EV) have been isolated from NMSC arising in OTRs recently [30]. Mixed viral infections consisting of HPV types from the cutaneous and mucosal families of HPV in combination with EV HPV types have been identified frequently in post-transplantation SCC [31].

The association of human herpesvirus 8 (HHV8) with AIDS-related and most other forms of KS is well known [32,33]. More recently, HHV8 infection has been shown to confer a significantly increased risk of KS among OTRs. In one study of kidney transplant recipients, nearly one quarter of patients who developed KS were HHV8 seropositive before transplantation, suggesting that reactivation of a latent viral infection might be central to the pathogenesis of this disease [34].

## Relationship of immunosuppression to skin cancer

Pharmacologic immunosuppression, required for long-term organ graft survival, increases the risk of cancer (and specifically skin cancer) by interfering with immunosurveillance and by augmenting viral proliferation. The risk of cutaneous malignancy is thought to show a dose- and duration-dependent relationship with overall immunosuppression [4,10]. Innumerable studies, many of which are retrospective, have attempted to define the relative risk of skin cancer conferred by individual agents or commonly used multi-drug regimens. More data are available on regimens containing combinations of corticosteroids, cyclosporine, and azathioprine than any of the newer agents including tacrolimus, mycophenolate mofetil, and sirolimus. Cross-study heterogeneity makes it difficult to synthesize the available literature into a cohesive set of clinical guidelines. Nevertheless, there are emerging trends.

Cyclosporine has been shown to confer substantial in vitro and in vivo malignant potential to cells [35]. A recent multicenter, multinational prospective cohort study of 1252 patients who had psoriasis who were treated with cyclosporine (average dose 3 mg/kg, mean duration 1.9 years) demonstrated a six-fold increase in the incidence of NMSC [36]. Cyclosporine doses used in OTRs can exceed those used in psoriasis by a factor of 3 to 4, and these results are consistent with many—though not all—published reports of cyclosporine use in transplant recipients [6,18,37–40]. Of note, the rate of SCC exceeded that of BCC by a factor of 3, similar to the ratio observed in OTRs. Studies of anti-metabolite therapy suggest that azathioprine-based therapy might also increase the risk of skin cancer [18]. Few data are available regarding the relative risk of mycophenolate mofetil, which might be less carcinogenic than cyclosporine or azathioprine [18].

There is preliminary evidence to suggest that sirolimus might partially mitigate the potent carcinogenic effects of cyclosporine, although prospective studies with long-term follow-up are currently lacking [41–44]. Fifteen kidney transplant recipients who had biopsy-proven KS underwent conversion from cyclosporine to sirolimus therapy after excisional biopsy of the lesion. Three months after cessation of cyclosporine, all cutaneous KS lesions had resolved. Before initiating sirolimus, the expression of vascular endothelial growth factor (VEGF) was shown to be increased in both lesional KS cells and apparently normal perilesional skin. Sirolimus is known to inhibit VEGF production and the response of vascular endothelial cells to VEGF, suggesting that it might have anti-tumor activity in KS [41–44].

### Risk factors for skin cancer

Many risk factors have been identified in OTRs that appear to confer increased susceptibility to skin cancer. Older age (>60 years) has been associated with a 19.8-fold risk of developing SCC compared with younger age [7]. Fair complexion [13,45], blue eyes [46], male gender [47], and human leukocyte antigen (HLA)-DR7 homozygosity [16] have also been associated with increased risk of skin cancer in OTRs. In selected cases the etiology of end-organ disease necessitating organ transplantation might confer a significant increase in the risk of post-transplant skin cancer. Antecedent polycystic kidney disease in kidney transplant recipients (RR 1.65, $P < 0.001$) and cholestatic liver disease in liver transplant recipients (RR 1.80, $P = 0.03$) were significantly more common among individuals who developed cutaneous malignancy in the post-transplant period [48].

### Skin cancer risk stratification before transplantation

Before undergoing organ transplantation, candidates should receive a comprehensive dermatologic history and full-body skin examination with emphasis on skin cancer. A risk profile should be created for each individual to include detailed documentation of the following: history of skin cancer, pre-malignant lesions including actinic keratoses, and porokeratoses (well-demarcated red to brown plaques with a characteristic moat of scale that are more prevalent and more commonly associated with NMSC in the transplant population), and viral warts or other evidence of HPV infection. Evidence of significant photodamage (Glogau types 3 and 4), occupational or recreational sun exposure or sunburns, family history of skin cancer (particularly melanoma), skin phototype (fair, freckled, and easily burned skin, Fitzpatrick skin types I–III), blue, green, or hazel eyes, red or blonde hair, diffuse freckling, solar lentigines (sun spots) or multiple nevi (>50) [49], and CD4 lymphocytopenia should also be evaluated.

A full-body skin (including the genitalia) and lymph node examination is indicated initially on an annual basis and more frequently for patients who have increased risk.

All transplant candidates should be screened for pre-existing medical conditions that could cause significant morbidity and premature mortality following transplantation. Potential candidates who have a history of skin cancer pose a particular challenge. Because the risks of recurrence and metastasis of prior skin cancer and the development of de novo carcinomas varies widely, a case-by-case assessment of individual patient risks is warranted.

The morbidity and mortality of prior skin cancers is most closely related to the histologic subtype of tumor. The risk of metastasis of BCC is exceedingly low, and recurrent locally invasive disease can usually be treated by conventional means (Fig. 2). Morbidity from BCC is related more to the propensity for new primary BCCs to develop in the post-transplant period. Except for the rare occurrence of metastatic disease, history of BCC should not be a contraindication for transplantation [50].

Squamous cell carcinoma is one of the most common and potentially fatal cutaneous malignancies arising in OTRs. Mortality has been attributed largely to a two-fold increase in the risk of metastasis (7% versus 3.6%) in OTRs compared with the general population [21,51]. Low-risk lesions should not affect the eligibility of candidates for transplantation, whereas a recent history (within 3 years) of high-risk primary lesions should be evaluated carefully with consultation by a transplant dermatologist or Mohs surgeon before transplantation. Metastatic SCC is associated with a poor prognosis among OTRs, in whom the 3- and 5-year survival rate is 56% and 34%, respectively (Fig. 3) [20]. As such, some authors propose that evaluation of potential candidates for transplantation should be delayed for 3 to 5 years when there is a history of high-risk primary, recurrent, or metastatic SCC [50].

Melanoma is becoming quite common in the general population, with more than 55,000 cases diagnosed in the United States annually [52]. Despite the rising incidence of this disease, case fatality (the number of deaths attributable to melanoma among affected individuals) is low relative to many other systemic malignancies. Current estimates for the 5-year survival rate among individuals who have invasive melanoma is 80% to 85% [53]. An additional 45,000 cases of in situ melanoma are diagnosed annually, for which the theoretical rate of metastasis is zero. Such cases should not preclude transplantation [50]. Individuals who have superficially invasive tumors (<1 mm thick) without ulceration have a 5-year survival rate of 95%, and individuals who have a remote history (at least 5 years prior) of melanoma should be considered for transplantation [53]. Patients who have thick primary melanomas, or locally recurrent or metastatic disease (Fig. 4) have a substantially poorer prognosis (5-year survival rate of roughly 50%). The propensity for melanoma to recur in the setting of immunosuppression despite years of remission is well recognized by the transplant community. In

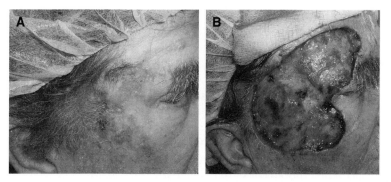

Fig. 2. (*A*) Right temple showing an ill-defined pink sclerotic plaque of BCC. (*B*) the Mohs surgery defect demonstrating the ill-defined clinical borders of the tumor.

only rare, life-saving circumstances are organs from donors who have a history of melanoma recovered for transplantation.

A recent history (within 3 years) of uncommon cutaneous malignancies including MCC, KS, atypical fibroxanthoma, dermatofibrosarcoma protuberans, sebaceous carcinoma, eccrine/syringomatous carcinoma, microcystic adnexal carcinoma, and extramammary Paget's disease should be carefully evaluated in consultation with a transplant dermatologist [50].

## Prevention of skin cancer

Organ transplant recipients and candidates for organ transplantation need to be formally educated verbally, in writing, and ideally by viewing an instructional video presentation regarding the risk of skin cancer in the post-transplant period. Principles of primary prevention, early detection, and regular follow-up care should be integrated. Emphasis should be placed on understanding the association of skin cancer with exposure to UVR. OTRs should be taught the signs and symptoms of skin cancer with particular attention paid to new or changing lesions that are persistent over the course of weeks to months. The authors advocate monthly, systematic,

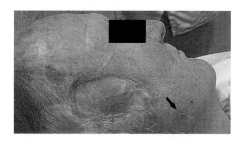

Fig. 3. Right cheek showing a subtle pink plaque of in-transit metastasis of SCC and the surgical scar superiorly where the primary tumor arose.

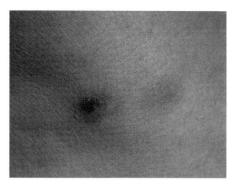

Fig. 4. Flank showing an ulcerated nodule of amelanotic melanoma and the discontiguous erythematous papule representing in-transit metastasis.

thorough self skin and lymph node examinations using a partner or mirrors to adequately image all areas. The utility of this exercise has not been studied in the transplant population but it is routinely advised in the general population among individuals who have a history of NMSC, atypical nevi, or a personal or family history of melanoma.

The importance of sunscreen and lip balm that have broad spectrum UVA and UVB protection optimally containing zinc, titanium, mexoryl, or avobenzone preparations and a high sun protection factor (>30) is underscored. In addition, sun-protective clothing (long sleeves, pants, and a wide brimmed hat) and avoidance of mid-day sun (generally from 10:00 AM to 4:00 PM), when exposure to UVR from the sun is most intense, should also be emphasized. Regular follow-up with a dermatologist for full skin examinations will promote early detection and treatment and provide an opportunity for ongoing patient education and reinforcement of the concern for the development of skin cancer. The hazards of tanning bed use should be strongly reinforced because currently there are compelling data that demonstrate significantly increased risks of BCC, SCC, and melanoma in some cases after surprisingly modest exposures to UVR in a tanning bed [54,55].

There is evidence to suggest that skin cancer prevention initiatives have a measurable (though modest) benefit toward reducing risk. One study reported sun protective behaviors among OTRs including always applying sunscreen increased from 6% to 37% in the post-transplant period [56]. The occurrence of skin cancer was significantly higher among individuals who did not practice sun safety.

Awareness of the importance of sun protection among OTRs who receive regular education might be higher at institutions where dermatologists are actively involved in the transplant services clinician team [57]. Ongoing education is necessary to reinforce the principles of skin cancer prevention in OTRs, for whom frequent visits with transplant physicians and management of symptomatic co-morbid medical conditions might dominate [58].

## Management of skin cancer

The most important step in the management of cutaneous malignancy in the post-transplant setting is the identification of high-risk lesions that warrant aggressive treatment.

SCC, the most commonly occurring histologic subtype of skin cancer, is often a high-risk lesion in the setting of immunosuppression [21,59].

Criteria for high-risk SCC have been outlined by the International Transplant Skin Cancer Collaborative (ITSCC) (Box 1) [60].

Diagnosis of a high-risk skin cancer warrants additional workup for evidence of metastasis. A physical examination must include a careful inspection of the primary lesion for evidence of satellite or in-transit metastases that might be apparent at the periphery as well as a thorough palpation of lymph nodes for evidence of regional metastasis.

Detailed algorithms for the management of pre-malignant and malignant lesions can be found in the guidelines established by the ITSCC [60]. There is ample evidence that Mohs micrographic surgery offers the highest cure rate for SCC and should be strongly considered for any high-risk tumor. The advantage of the Mohs technique, which uses horizontal en-face sectioning of fresh frozen tissue blocks, is derived from the ability to achieve 100%

---

**Box 1. Criteria for high-risk SCC of the skin**

Location (independent of size) including tumors arising on the
  central face, eyelids and periorbital skin, eyebrows, nose, lips,
  ears, chin and mandible, pre- and post- auricular skin, temples,
  genitalia, hands, and feet
Size >10 mm arising on the cheeks, forehead, neck, or scalp
  or >20 mm arising on the trunk and extremities
Rapid growth
Ulceration
Indistinct clinical borders
Aggressive histology defined by the presence of extension of the
  tumor into the subcutaneous fat and/or >4 mm in depth,
  perineural invasion or inflammation, perivascular or
  intravascular invasion, single-cell invasion, or cytologic
  features of poor differentiation
Recurrence in the site of prior treatment
Occurrence in a scar or area of chronic inflammation
The presence of satellite lesions
The presence of multiple SCCs
Clinical, radiographic, or histologic evidence of lymph node
  involvement

margin control by way of direct observation of the entire specimen (epidermis, dermis, and underlying tissues) surrounding the lesion. Intraoperative vertical sectioning of fresh frozen tissue or traditional bread loaf sectioning of paraffin-embedded tissue blocks permit evaluation of less than 5% of the specimen margin and can result in an erroneous determination of clear margins, particularly among poorly differentiated and infiltrative tumors.

For these reasons, standard excision or wide local excision might be inadequate in the treatment of SCC arising in OTRs caused by the common presence of subclinical tumor extension [61]. Surgical excision with a 6 mm margin of normal skin beyond any surrounding erythema and postoperative margin assessment of permanent tissue sectioning might produce adequate clearance rates in the presence of subclinical microscopic tumor extension if intraoperative evaluation of frozen sections is not available [62].

SCC demonstrating a less aggressive histologic pattern can also be treated with destructive methods including cryosurgery and electrodesiccation and curettage, as well as excision and Mohs micrographic surgery. Primary treatment with radiotherapy might be indicated in OTRs who have inoperable tumors or in patients who are poor surgical candidates because of the presence of significant co-morbidities. Radiation can also be considered as an adjunctive therapy when clear surgical margins are not attainable or when there is histologic evidence of perineural invasion or inflammation. In cases of SCC with perineural involvement, adjuvant radiation might be particularly beneficial, even with clear surgical margins [63]. The efficacy of radiation is limited by the inability to evaluate histologically the margins of the treatment area for the presence of tumor. In addition, because OTRs tend to develop areas of confluent skin dysplasia it is difficult often to identify the clinical border of the tumor [60].

The presence of in-transit metastasis warrants additional workup to evaluate for distant metastasis. Aggressive treatment, usually with Mohs micrographic surgery or wide excision followed by adjuvant radiation, is generally indicated. Evidence-based guidelines regarding the use of sentinel lymph node biopsy and specific radiographic imaging modalities (eg, PET, CT, and MRI) are currently lacking.

Pre-malignant squamous lesions including actinic keratoses, porokeratoses, and verrucae can be treated with topical therapy (including 5-fluorouracil, imiquimod, or diclofenac) or destructive methods (including cryotherapy, curettage, or electrosurgery). Consideration for adjuvant treatment in patients who have multiple lesions and a field effect would include photodynamic therapy, topical retinoids, chemical peels, dermabrasion, and resurfacing with the Nd:Erbium or $CO_2$ lasers. A recent survey of 25 transplant dermatologists revealed that most use 5-fluorouracil and half use topical retinoids to treat actinic keratoses [64]. Nearly all respondents use cryosurgery for warts and actinic keratoses. All respondents recommend Mohs micrographic surgery for skin cancer when indicated and nearly all recommend excision with wide margins when Mohs is not indicated or unavailable.

## Dose reduction of immunosuppressive agents

Definitive evidence-based data are lacking to assist the transplant physician when considering whether or not to reduce the level of pharmacologic immunosuppression in patients who are developing skin cancers and consequently accept an increased risk of organ rejection. Intuitively, the management of a low-risk skin cancer should differ from that of a life-threatening tumor burden with severely impaired quality of life. It has been observed generally that reducing the level of immunosuppression results in a concomitant mitigation of the number of new skin cancers and of the aggressive behavior that is typical of cutaneous malignancies among OTRs [65,66]. Additional support for the causal relationship between iatrogenic immunosuppression and cutaneous malignancy are observations that post-transplant KS and lymphoproliferative disorders often remit spontaneously following immune reconstitution. The viral etiology associated with these malignancies (HHV8 with KS and Epstein-Barr virus with post-transplant lymphoproliferative disorder) suggests that restoring immune surveillance and antiviral immunity might be critical in arresting carcinogenesis in this population [67].

The ITSCC has proposed broad guidelines for dose reduction by recommending the minimum level of immunosuppression required to safely maintain graft function [60]. Based on significant clinical experience and observational data it has been suggested that a reduction of immunosuppression is indicated in the setting of high risk-tumors, multiple local recurrences of aggressive SCC, metastases, or catastrophic carcinogenesis with more than 100 primary tumors per year [21,65,68,69]. A prospective randomized study of low-dose (75–125 ng/mL) cyclosporine compared with a normal dose (150–250 ng/mL) in kidney transplant recipients over 5 years demonstrated significantly lower risk of skin cancer in the low-dose group; no difference in subject or graft survival was noted despite more frequent symptoms of graft rejection in this group [70]. Azathioprine and cyclosporine are often targeted for reduction or discontinuation because of the association with skin cancer development. Sirolimus and mycophenolate mofetil might preserve graft survival and might be less carcinogenic agents, although evidence-based guidelines are not yet available [24].

A recent survey of the ITSCC [71] reported a unanimous consensus that mild reduction of immunosuppression is appropriate for kidney transplant recipients who are developing 2 to 25 NMSCs per year or stage IA melanoma, for which 3-year mortality does not exceed 2%. Moderate impairment in the quality of life because of the burden of skin cancer can be observed in this subgroup of patients. Moderate reduction was considered to be indicated for patients who developed more than 25 skin cancers per year or for specific malignancies (including high-risk SCC, MCC, and stage IIA–B melanoma), for which the 3-year mortality rate is approximately 10% to 25%. Severe reduction was recommended for life-threatening skin cancers including metastatic SCC, stage IIC/III or IV melanoma, MCC (any stage), and visceral KS, for which the 3-year mortality rate exceeds 50%.

In general, metastatic potential of individual skin cancers was a stronger indication for aggressive dose reduction than quality of life impairment. The task force also recommended that all OTRs who have stable graft function be considered for prophylactic reduction of immunosuppression as early as 1 to 2 years after transplantation in an effort to balance the importance of graft preservation with the risk of cutaneous malignancy [60]. More aggressive dose reduction was advised for kidney transplant recipients for whom dialysis was considered a sustainable alternative in the event of graft failure compared with heart and liver transplant recipients, for whom graft failure is likely fatal. Liver recipients were considered to be more likely than heart recipients to successfully wean off immunosuppressant medications, and liver allografts were thought to have comparatively lower immunogenicity and a greater capacity to tolerate episodes of rejection [60]. Recommendations for dose reduction among liver transplant recipients were therefore more aggressive than those for heart transplant recipients.

### Chemoprevention with retinoids

All OTRs who begin to develop progressive carcinogenesis should be evaluated for chemoprophylaxis with a systemic retinoid such as acitretin accompanied by appropriate laboratory testing. The use of systemic retinoids for chemoprevention of NMSC was initially studied in patients who had a predisposition to cutaneous malignancy arising from genetic defects in DNA repair machinery. Xeroderma pigmentosum and nevoid BCC syndrome are two genodermatoses (genetically determined skin disorders) in which the risk of UVR-induced skin cancer is significant and a common cause of premature mortality in affected individuals [72–74].

The effect of systemic retinoids, which act to promote keratinocyte maturation and apoptosis of damaged cells as well as epidermal thinning and keratinization, has been shown to reduce to the occurrence of skin cancer. The suppressive effect is transient, however, and rapid recrudescence might be observed upon cessation of therapy, although continued protective effects have been noted in some patients up to 8 years following treatment [75–77].

Similar studies of systemic retinoids in pharmacologically immunosuppressed OTRs have been performed [78]. Treatment with oral acitretin (25–30 mg daily) has been shown to substantially reduce the development of keratotic lesions including actinic keratoses and SCC, particularly among OTRs who have a prior history of skin cancer [75,79]. Similar relapse rates were observed upon cessation of therapy and nearly half of patients experienced significant toxicity, requiring adjustment of the dosing frequency to 25 mg every other day.

In an effort to increase patient tolerability of acitretin, lower doses of 0.3 mg/kg/d have been studied [76]. A marked reduction in the occurrence of skin cancer was observed over a 4-year course of treatment. Shorter courses might not be effective in reducing the number of SCCs, however [80].

Side effects of oral retinoids commonly include xerosis (dry skin), hair loss, mucocutaneous irritation and dryness, and palmar–plantar desquamation [81]. Laboratory abnormalities including liver transaminitis and hyperlipidemia (particularly hypertriglyceridemia) are largely dose-dependent but might occur idiosyncratically in susceptible individuals at very low doses. The association of hyperlipidemia and ischemic cardiovascular events or pancreatitis necessitates close collaboration between the transplant physician and the prescribing dermatologist. Musculoskeletal side effects, including myalgias, arthralgias, and (rarely) skeletal hyperostosis (diffuse idiopathic skeletal hyperostosis) can occur. There is some suggestion that oral retinoids might be associated with osteoporosis, a significant concern in OTRs who often receive long-term treatment with corticosteroids that are independently strongly associated with osteoporosis [82,83]. Headache, drowsiness, loss of night vision, peripheral sensorimotor neuropathy, and benign intracranial hypertension (pseudotumor cerebri) have been reported [84]. Reversible hair loss is expected in approximately 20% of patients. Other nonspecific symptoms including malaise, nausea, and sweating can occur. Despite reports of suicidality and mood disorders in patients taking isotretinoin, another systemic retinoid, there have been no such reports in patients taking acitretin. Because of the frequent side effect of xerophthalmia and the risk of serious structural corneal damage including ulceration, infection, decreased vision, and loss of vision, the laser-assisted in situ keratomileusis (LASIK) operation for vision correction is generally contraindicated in patients taking systemic retinoids until 6 months after the cessation of treatment; similarly, patient screening for a recent history of the LASIK procedure should be performed before initiating oral retinoids [85].

Notably, acitretin, along with other systemic retinoids, are pregnancy category X and are known to be teratogenic in pregnant females. Although there is no compelling evidence to suggest that systemic retinoids confer a significant risk of teratogenicity through transmission in paternal seminal fluid, patients should be strongly counseled that definitive studies are lacking [86]. Alcohol consumption concomitant with the use of acitretin is known to produce an active metabolite (etretinate) that has a significantly longer half-life (120 days versus 2 days) and would effectively require a 2- to 3-year post-treatment holiday to eliminate the risk of teratogenicity. Absolute cessation of alcohol use is recommended.

Although the theoretical risk has been postulated, there have been no convincing data demonstrating any increased risk of graft rejection associated with an immunostimulatory effect of an oral retinoid. The effect of systemic retinoids on wound healing has not been fully delineated, and results of preliminary studies examining the tendency toward hypertrophic granulation tissue, poor wound healing, and increased scarring have been mixed [87,88]. There appears to be no increased risk of postoperative wound infection or dehiscence. Ultimately, decisions regarding surgical management of cutaneous malignancies should be made independently from consideration of systemic retinoid therapy.

The use of topical retinoids also has been shown to reduce the clinical appearance of actinic keratoses in OTRs, but long-term treatment might be required [89,90]. No long-term studies of topical retinoids on the development of NMSC in OTRs have been performed.

Recommendations for OTRs who have multiple actinic keratoses include topical tretinoin at increasing concentrations and frequency (as tolerated) until the desired clinical outcome is achieved. Adjunctive therapy for thick or recalcitrant actinic keratoses might include topical 5-fluorouracil, topical diclofenac, imiquimod, topical delta aminolevulinic acid ($\delta$ALA) photodynamic therapy, chemical peels, and curettage [91–93].

## Frequency of follow-up care

In general, OTRs might need more frequent follow-up care compared with non-immunosuppressed patients [21]. The importance of an initial full-body skin examination by a dermatologist cannot be overemphasized. Subsequently, patients who have a low risk for skin cancer should receive a full skin examination annually by a dermatologist. More frequent follow-up care is required for patients who have a history of premalignant or malignant skin lesions. A low threshold for monthly or bimonthly visits should be maintained and the frequency extended only when the occurrence of new lesions and the progression of low-risk lesions has been demonstrated (typically over the course of 1–3 years) to be flat or slow.

## Interdisciplinary approach

The development of a multidisciplinary approach to providing comprehensive care for OTRs at risk for skin cancer has been adopted at many institutions. The rationale for creating a specialty clinic is based upon the need to provide high-quality care that is proactive and efficient [94]. Because high-risk OTRs have the propensity to develop multiple cutaneous malignancies over a short period of time, the capacity to expedite diagnosis and implement an interdisciplinary treatment plan is critical in patients whose tumor burden might become life-threatening. Among lower-risk OTRs, the opportunity for primary prevention, patient education, early detection, chemoprophylaxis, and to reduce morbidity from cutaneous malignancy is enhanced by an interdisciplinary paradigm.

Representation from departments or divisions including dermatology, dermatologic surgery, subspecialty medical and surgical transplant services, facial plastic surgery, oculoplastic and head and neck surgery, radiation and medical oncology, psychiatry, endocrinology, and infectious disease and cardiovascular medicine, among others, is essential for optimal care of the transplant patient. A multidisciplinary model for delivering health care is needed in which a network of physician specialists maintains direct lines of communication and provides timely access to medical services by reserving appointment slots for OTRs who require comprehensive medical services [94].

## Changing emphasis over time

More than one quarter of deaths occurring at least 4 years after transplantation are attributable to skin cancer, so it is imperative that following the post-operative period and stabilization of the immunosuppressant regimen, increased emphasis be placed on diagnosis and treatment of skin cancer in an effort to reduce morbidity and mortality from this disease. Vigilance by an experienced clinician and frequent follow-up care is necessary to identify the incipient stages of rapid tumor development and to act decisively by initiating chemosuppressive therapy with oral retinoids when appropriate. The importance of detailed written and photographic documentation in the medical record and continuity of care with the same clinician should be underscored. Careful consideration should be given to the frequency of new lesions and the risk profile of individual premalignant and malignant lesions. High-risk OTRs tend to enter a rapidly escalating phase of unstable carcinogenesis in which the occurrence of malignant lesions can quickly become difficult to manage with conventional therapies. The precision required to execute an efficacious management plan in these complex situations highlights the need for a facile multidisciplinary team of knowledgeable and dedicated clinicians.

## References

[1] Moloney FJ, Keane S, O'Kelly P, et al. The impact of skin disease following renal transplantation on quality of life. Br J Dermatol 2005;153(3):574–8.
[2] Penn I. Occurrence of cancers in immunosuppressed organ transplant recipients. Clin Transpl 1994;7:99–109.
[3] Sheil AG, Disney AP, Mathew TH, et al. De novo malignancy emerges as a major cause of morbidity and late failure in renal transplantation. Transplant Proc 1993;25(1 Pt 2):1383–4.
[4] Moloney FJ, Comber H, O'Lorcain P, et al. A population-based study of skin cancer incidence and prevalence in renal transplant recipients. Br J Dermatol 2006;154(3):498–504.
[5] Blohme I, Larko O. Skin lesions in renal transplant patients after 10–23 years of immunosuppressive therapy. Acta Derm Venereol 1990;70(6):491–4.
[6] Bouwes Bavinck JN, Hardie DR, Green A, et al. The risk of skin cancer in renal transplant recipients in Queensland, Australia. A follow-up study. Transplantation 1996;61(5):715–21.
[7] Jensen P, Hansen S, Moller B, et al. Skin cancer in kidney and heart transplant recipients and different long-term immunosuppressive therapy regimens. J Am Acad Dermatol 1999;40 (2 Pt 1):177–86.

[8] Adami J, Gabel H, Lindelof B, et al. Cancer risk following organ transplantation: a nation-wide cohort study in Sweden. Br J Cancer 2003;89(7):1221–7.

[9] Otley CC, Pittelkow MR. Skin cancer in liver transplant recipients. Liver Transpl 2000;6(3):253–62.

[10] Ulrich C, Schmook T, Sachse MM, et al. Comparative epidemiology and pathogenic factors for nonmelanoma skin cancer in organ transplant patients. Dermatol Surg 2004;30(4 Pt 2):622–7.

[11] Ramsay HM, Fryer AA, Hawley CM, et al. Non-melanoma skin cancer risk in the Queensland renal transplant population. Br J Dermatol 2002;147(5):950–6.

[12] Staples MP, Elwood M, Burton RC, et al. Non-melanoma skin cancer in Australia: the 2002 national survey and trends since 1985. Med J Aust 2006;184(1):6–10.

[13] Espana A, Redondo P, Fernandez AL, et al. Skin cancer in heart transplant recipients. J Am Acad Dermatol 1995;32(3):458–65.

[14] Webb MC, Compton F, Andrews PA, et al. Skin tumours posttransplantation: a retrospective analysis of 28 years' experience at a single centre. Transplant Proc 1997;29(1–2):828–30.

[15] Euvrard S, Kanitakis J, Pouteil-Noble C, et al. Comparative epidemiologic study of premalignant and malignant epithelial cutaneous lesions developing after kidney and heart transplantation. J Am Acad Dermatol 1995;33(2 Pt 1):222–9.

[16] Ong CS, Keogh AM, Kossard S, et al. Skin cancer in Australian heart transplant recipients. J Am Acad Dermatol 1999;40(1):27–34.

[17] Hollenbeak CS, Todd MM, Billingsley EM, et al. Increased incidence of melanoma in renal transplantation recipients. Cancer 2005;104(9):1962–7.

[18] Kasiske BL, Snyder JJ, Gilbertson DT, et al. Cancer after kidney transplantation in the United States. Am J Transplant 2004;4(6):905–13.

[19] Penn I, First MR. Merkel's cell carcinoma in organ recipients: report of 41 cases. Transplantation 1999;68(11):1717–21.

[20] Martinez JC, Otley CC, Stasko T, et al. Defining the clinical course of metastatic skin cancer in organ transplant recipients: a multicenter collaborative study. Arch Dermatol 2003;139(3):301–6.

[21] Berg D, Otley CC. Skin cancer in organ transplant recipients: epidemiology, pathogenesis, and management. J Am Acad Dermatol 2002;47(1):1–17; quiz 8–20.

[22] Penn I. Tumors after renal and cardiac transplantation. Hematol Oncol Clin N Am 1993;7(2):431–45.

[23] Lewis KG, Weinstock MA. Nonmelanoma skin cancer mortality (1988–2000): the Rhode Island follow-back study. Arch Dermatol 2004;140(7):837–42.

[24] Buell JF, Gross TG, Woodle ES. Malignancy after transplantation. Transplantation 2005;80(2 Suppl):S254–64.

[25] Grossman D, Leffell DJ. The molecular basis of nonmelanoma skin cancer: new understanding. Arch Dermatol 1997;133(10):1263–70.

[26] Brash DE, Ziegler A, Jonason AS, et al. Sunlight and sunburn in human skin cancer: p53, apoptosis, and tumor promotion. J Investig Dermatol Symp Proc 1996;1(2):136–42.

[27] Carucci JA. Cutaneous oncology in organ transplant recipients: meeting the challenge of squamous cell carcinoma. J Invest Dermatol 2004;123(5):809–16.

[28] Parrish JA. Immunosuppression, skin cancer, and ultraviolet A radiation. N Engl J Med 2005;353(25):2712–3.

[29] Euvrard S, Chardonnet Y, Pouteil-Noble C, et al. Association of skin malignancies with various and multiple carcinogenic and noncarcinogenic human papillomaviruses in renal transplant recipients. Cancer 1993;72(7):2198–206.

[30] Harwood CA, Surentheran T, Sasieni P, et al. Increased risk of skin cancer associated with the presence of epidermodysplasia verruciformis human papillomavirus types in normal skin. Br J Dermatol 2004;150(5):949–57.

[31] Purdie KJ, Surentheran T, Sterling JC, et al. Human papillomavirus gene expression in cutaneous squamous cell carcinomas from immunosuppressed and immunocompetent individuals. J Invest Dermatol 2005;125(1):98–107.

[32] Chang Y, Cesarman E, Pessin MS, et al. Identification of herpesvirus-like DNA sequences in AIDS-associated Kaposi's sarcoma. Science 1994;266(5192):1865–9.

[33] Schwartz RA. Kaposi's sarcoma: an update. J Surg Oncol 2004;87(3):146–51.

[34] Cattani P, Capuano M, Graffeo R, et al. Kaposi's sarcoma associated with previous human herpesvirus 8 infection in kidney transplant recipients. J Clin Microbiol 2001; 39(2):506–8.

[35] Durando B, Reichel J. The relative effects of different systemic immunosuppressives on skin cancer development in organ transplant patients. Dermatol Ther 2005;18(1):1–11.

[36] Paul CF, Ho VC, McGeown C, et al. Risk of malignancies in psoriasis patients treated with cyclosporine: a 5 y cohort study. J Invest Dermatol 2003;120(2):211–6.

[37] Hiesse C, Larue JR, Kriaa F, et al. Incidence and type of malignancies occurring after renal transplantation in conventionally and in cyclosporine-treated recipients: single-center analysis of a 20-year period in 1600 patients. Transplant Proc 1995;27(4):2450–1.

[38] Penn I. Cancers in cyclosporine-treated vs azathioprine-treated patients. Transplant Proc 1996;28(2):876–8.

[39] Glover MT, Deeks JJ, Raftery MJ, et al. Immunosuppression and risk of non-melanoma skin cancer in renal transplant recipients. Lancet 1997;349(9049):398.

[40] Jensen P, Hansen S, Moller B, et al. Are renal transplant recipients on CsA-based immuno-suppressive regimens more likely to develop skin cancer than those on azathioprine and prednisolone? Transplant Proc 1999;31(1–2):1120.

[41] Kreis H, Oberbauer R, Campistol JM, et al. Long-term benefits with sirolimus-based therapy after early cyclosporine withdrawal. J Am Soc Nephrol 2004;15(3):809–17.

[42] Kahan BD, Yakupoglu YK, Schoenberg L, et al. Low incidence of malignancy among sirolimus/cyclosporine-treated renal transplant recipients. Transplantation 2005;80(6): 749–58.

[43] Euvrard S, Ulrich C, Lefrancois N. Immunosuppressants and skin cancer in transplant patients: focus on rapamycin. Dermatol Surg 2004;30(4 Pt 2):628–33.

[44] Mathew T, Kreis H, Friend P. Two-year incidence of malignancy in sirolimus-treated renal transplant recipients: results from five multicenter studies. Clin Transplant 2004;18(4): 446–9.

[45] Lindelof B, Granath F, Dal H, et al. Sun habits in kidney transplant recipients with skin cancer: a case-control study of possible causative factors. Acta Derm Venereol 2003;83(3): 189–93.

[46] Lampros TD, Cobanoglu A, Parker F, et al. Squamous and basal cell carcinoma in heart transplant recipients. J Heart Lung Transplant 1998;17(6):586–91.

[47] Naldi L, Fortina AB, Lovati S, et al. Risk of nonmelanoma skin cancer in Italian organ transplant recipients. A registry-based study. Transplantation 2000;70(10):1479–84.

[48] Otley CC, Cherikh WS, Salasche SJ, et al. Skin cancer in organ transplant recipients: effect of pretransplant end-organ disease. J Am Acad Dermatol 2005;53(5):783–90.

[49] Garbe C, Buttner P, Weiss J, et al. Associated factors in the prevalence of more than 50 common melanocytic nevi, atypical melanocytic nevi, and actinic lentigines: multicenter case-control study of the Central Malignant Melanoma Registry of the German Dermatological Society. J Invest Dermatol 1994;102(5):700–5.

[50] Otley CC, Hirose R, Salasche SJ. Skin cancer as a contraindication to organ transplantation. Am J Transplant 2005;5(9):2079–84.

[51] Chuang TY, Popescu NA, Su WP, et al. Squamous cell carcinoma. A population-based incidence study in Rochester. Minn Arch Dermatol 1990;126(2):185–8.

[52] Jemal A, Tiwari RC, Murray T, et al. Cancer statistics, 2004. CA Cancer J Clin 2004;54(1): 8–29.

[53] Balch CM, Buzaid AC, Soong SJ, et al. Final version of the American Joint Committee on Cancer staging system for cutaneous melanoma. J Clin Oncol 2001;19(16):3635–48.

[54] Karagas MR, Stannard VA, Mott LA, et al. Use of tanning devices and risk of basal cell and squamous cell skin cancers. J Natl Cancer Inst 2002;94(3):224–6.

[55] Westerdahl J, Olsson H, Masback A, et al. Use of sunbeds or sunlamps and malignant melanoma in southern Sweden. Am J Epidemiol 1994;140(8):691–9.

[56] Moloney FJ, Almarzouqi E, O'Kelly P, et al. Sunscreen use before and after transplantation and assessment of risk factors associated with skin cancer development in renal transplant recipients. Arch Dermatol 2005;141(8):978–82.

[57] Mahe E, Morelon E, Fermanian J, et al. Renal-transplant recipients and sun protection. Transplantation 2004;78(5):741–4.

[58] Cowen EW, Billingsley EM. Awareness of skin cancer by kidney transplant patients. J Am Acad Dermatol 1999;40(5 Pt 1):697–701.

[59] Rowe DE, Carroll RJ, Day CL Jr. Prognostic factors for local recurrence, metastasis, and survival rates in squamous cell carcinoma of the skin, ear, and lip. Implications for treatment modality selection. J Am Acad Dermatol 1992;26(6):976–90.

[60] Stasko T, Brown MD, Carucci JA, et al. Guidelines for the management of squamous cell carcinoma in organ transplant recipients. Dermatol Surg 2004;30(4 Pt 2):642–50.

[61] Mehrany K, Byrd DR, Roenigk RK, et al. Lymphocytic infiltrates and subclinical epithelial tumor extension in patients with chronic leukemia and solid-organ transplantation. Dermatol Surg 2003;29(2):129–34.

[62] Brodland DG, Zitelli JA. Surgical margins for excision of primary cutaneous squamous cell carcinoma. J Am Acad Dermatol 1992;27(2 Pt 1):241–8.

[63] Lawrence N, Cottel WI. Squamous cell carcinoma of skin with perineural invasion. J Am Acad Dermatol 1994;31(1):30–3.

[64] Clayton AS, Stasko T. Treatment of nonmelanoma skin cancer in organ transplant recipients: review of responses to a survey. J Am Acad Dermatol 2003;49(3):413–6.

[65] Ramos HC, Reyes J, Abu-Elmagd K, et al. Weaning of immunosuppression in long-term liver transplant recipients. Transplantation 1995;59(2):212–7.

[66] Otley CC, Coldiron BM, Stasko T, et al. Decreased skin cancer after cessation of therapy with transplant-associated immunosuppressants. Arch Dermatol 2001;137(4):459–63.

[67] Otley CC, Maragh SL. Reduction of immunosuppression for transplant-associated skin cancer: rationale and evidence of efficacy. Dermatol Surg 2005;31(2):163–8.

[68] Euvrard S, Kanitakis J, Pouteil-Noble C, et al. Aggressive squamous cell carcinomas in organ transplant recipients. Transplant Proc 1995;27(2):1767–8.

[69] Moloney FJ, Kelly PO, Kay EW, et al. Maintenance versus reduction of immunosuppression in renal transplant recipients with aggressive squamous cell carcinoma. Dermatol Surg 2004; 30(4 Pt 2):674–8.

[70] Dantal J, Hourmant M, Cantarovich D, et al. Effect of long-term immunosuppression in kidney-graft recipients on cancer incidence: randomised comparison of two cyclosporin regimens. Lancet 1998;351(9103):623–8.

[71] Otley CC, Berg D, Ulrich C, et al. Reduction of immunosuppression for transplant-associated skin cancer: expert consensus survey. Br J Dermatol 2006;154(3):395–400.

[72] DiGiovanna JJ. Posttransplantation skin cancer: scope of the problem, management, and role for systemic retinoid chemoprevention. Transplant Proc 1998;30(6):2771–5 [discussion 6–8].

[73] Kraemer KH, DiGiovanna JJ, Moshell AN, et al. Prevention of skin cancer in xeroderma pigmentosum with the use of oral isotretinoin. N Engl J Med 1988;318(25):1633–7.

[74] Peck GL, DiGiovanna JJ, Sarnoff DS, et al. Treatment and prevention of basal cell carcinoma with oral isotretinoin. J Am Acad Dermatol 1988;19(1 Pt 2):176–85.

[75] Bavinck JN, Tieben LM, Van der Woude FJ, et al. Prevention of skin cancer and reduction of keratotic skin lesions during acitretin therapy in renal transplant recipients: a double-blind, placebo-controlled study. J Clin Oncol 1995;13(8):1933–8.

[76] McKenna DB, Murphy GM. Skin cancer chemoprophylaxis in renal transplant recipients: 5 years of experience using low-dose acitretin. Br J Dermatol 1999;140(4):656–60.

[77] Harwood CA, Leedham-Green M, Leigh IM, et al. Low-dose retinoids in the prevention of cutaneous squamous cell carcinomas in organ transplant recipients: a 16-year retrospective study. Arch Dermatol 2005;141(4):456–64.

[78] Chen K, Craig JC, Shumack S. Oral retinoids for the prevention of skin cancers in solid organ transplant recipients: a systematic review of randomized controlled trials. Br J Dermatol 2005;152(3):518–23.

[79] George R, Weightman W, Russ GR, et al. Acitretin for chemoprevention of non-melanoma skin cancers in renal transplant recipients. Australas J Dermatol 2002;43(4):269–73.

[80] de Sevaux RG, Smit JV, de Jong EM, et al. Acitretin treatment of premalignant and malignant skin disorders in renal transplant recipients: clinical effects of a randomized trial comparing two doses of acitretin. J Am Acad Dermatol 2003;49(3):407–12.

[81] Kovach BT, Sams HH, Stasko T. Systemic strategies for chemoprevention of skin cancers in transplant recipients. Clin Transplant 2005;19(6):726–34.

[82] DiGiovanna JJ, Sollitto RB, Abangan DL, et al. Osteoporosis is a toxic effect of long-term etretinate therapy. Arch Dermatol 1995;131(11):1263–7.

[83] Summey BT, Yosipovitch G. Glucocorticoid-induced bone loss in dermatologic patients: an update. Arch Dermatol 2006;142(1):82–90.

[84] Wakeline SH, Maibach HI. Handbook of systemic drug treatment in dermatology. London: Manson Publishing Ltd.; 2004.

[85] Miles S, McGlathery W, Abernathie B. The importance of screening for laser-assisted in situ keratomileusis operation (LASIK) before prescribing isotretinoin. J Am Acad Dermatol 2006;54(1):180–1.

[86] Geiger JM, Walker M. Is there a reproductive safety risk in male patients treated with acitretin (neotigason/soriatane? Dermatology 2002;205(2):105–7.

[87] Neuhaus IM, Tope WD. Practical retinoid chemoprophylaxis in solid organ transplant recipients. Dermatol Ther 2005;18(1):28–33.

[88] Tan SR, Tope WD. Effect of acitretin on wound healing in organ transplant recipients. Dermatol Surg 2004;30(4 Pt 2):667–73.

[89] Odom R. Managing actinic keratoses with retinoids. J Am Acad Dermatol 1998;39(2 Pt 3): S74–8.

[90] Euvrard S, Verschoore M, Touraine JL, et al. Topical retinoids for warts and keratoses in transplant recipients. Lancet 1992;340(8810):48–9.

[91] Dragieva G, Hafner J, Dummer R, et al. Topical photodynamic therapy in the treatment of actinic keratoses and Bowen's disease in transplant recipients. Transplantation 2004;77(1): 115–21.

[92] Brown VL, Atkins CL, Ghali L, et al. Safety and efficacy of 5% imiquimod cream for the treatment of skin dysplasia in high-risk renal transplant recipients: randomized, double-blind, placebo-controlled trial. Arch Dermatol 2005;141(8):985–93.

[93] Smith KJ, Germain M, Skelton H. Squamous cell carcinoma in situ (Bowen's disease) in renal transplant patients treated with 5% imiquimod and 5% 5-fluorouracil therapy. Dermatol Surg 2001;27(6):561–4.

[94] Otley CC. Organization of a specialty clinic to optimize the care of organ transplant recipients at risk for skin cancer. Dermatol Surg 2000;26(7):709–12.

SURGICAL
CLINICS OF
NORTH AMERICA

Surg Clin N Am 86 (2006) 1277–1296

# Tolerance, Xenotransplantation: Future Therapies

Matthew J. Weiss, MD, Choo Y. Ng, MD,
Joren C. Madsen, MD, DPhil*

*Transplantation Biology Research Center and Division of Cardiac Surgery,
Department of Surgery, Massachusetts General Hospital, Harvard Medical School,
55 Fruit Street, Boston, MA 02114, USA*

The two biggest problems with solid organ transplantation are the lack of enough organs to transplant and the limited survival of transplanted organs (and their recipients). This review focuses on two future therapies that could solve these problems, specifically, tolerance induction to permit long-term patient and graft survival, and xenotransplantation to provide an unlimited supply of donor organs.

## Problem 1: allografts and their recipients do not survive long enough

Heart transplant registry data for 1992 to 2003 [1] show that infection (35.2%) and acute rejection (12.5%) are the leading causes of cardiac transplant recipient death between day 31 and 1 year post transplant. After 5 years, chronic rejection (16% to 30%) and malignancy (24%) account for most cardiac recipient deaths. Similar statistics apply to recipients of most solid organ transplants. Chronic nonspecific pharmacologic immunosuppression, as currently practiced, is the root cause of all of these problems. Immunosuppressive drugs increase susceptibility to infection and malignancy, cause morbid drug-specific side effects, and permit or even contribute to chronic rejection [2]. The need for strategies that eliminate the use of

This work was supported in part by National Institute of Health grants from the National Institute of Allergy and Infectious Disease (PO1AI50157, PO1AI50157, U19AI066705) and the National Heart, Lung and Blood Institute (RO1HL054211, RO1HL67110, RO1HL071932).

* Corresponding author. Department of Surgery, Massachusetts General Hospital, 55 Fruit Street, Bullfinch 119, Boston, MA 02114.

*E-mail address:* madsen@helix.mgh.harvard.edu (J.C. Madsen).

long-term immunosuppression and that prevent chronic rejection is patently clear.

## Solution 1: transplantation tolerance

Transplantation tolerance can be defined as an acquired modification to the host immune system that leads to indefinite, drug-free, allograft survival with maintenance of full immunocompetence. For 50 years, tolerance, as first accomplished experimentally by Medawar and coworkers [3], has evoked the promise of indefinite, drug-free graft survival devoid of any major complications, including chronic rejection [4]. Medawar's team demonstrated that prenatal or neonatal mice inoculated with allogeneic antigens (splenocytes) were tolerant as adults to skin grafts from the same donor strain. The permanent survival of these skin grafts established the feasibility of organ transplantation and fostered the hope that tolerance could be achieved in adults. Since that time, at least 50 additional strategies for tolerance induction have been described [4]; however, they have all been relegated to the laboratory rodent until recently, when the deliberate induction of mixed lymphohematopoietic chimerism in human renal transplant recipients induced sustained allograft tolerance [5,6]. Although challenges remain in achieving reproducible, robust, and long-lasting tolerance in recipients of HLA disparate organs, there is cause for excitement in the field.

### Mechanisms of tolerance

To understand how transplantation tolerance is achieved, one must understand how self-tolerance is induced and maintained. Tolerance to self is a continuous process that prevents immune responses from developing against self antigens. It depends upon central and peripheral components. Central tolerance refers to tolerance generated within the thymus using mechanisms that delete or eliminate T cells (also called deletional tolerance). In brief, specialized antigen-presenting cells in the thymus cause immature T cells with a high affinity for self major histocompatibility complex (MHC) molecules to undergo programmed cell death or apoptosis. This process, referred to as negative selection, prevents autoimmunity by removing potentially autoreactive T cells.

Peripheral tolerance refers to extrathymic mechanisms that affect T cells that have escaped negative selection and emigrated from the thymus. There are several mechanisms by which peripheral tolerance occurs. The most dominant peripheral form of tolerance seems be mediated by specialized T cells, termed *regulatory cells* (T regs), which are able to suppress the responses of other activated T cells [7]. By regulating immune responses, they likely orchestrate beneficial immune responses and silence harmful ones. Although peripheral pathways are effective, it is unlikely that any of them independently leads to the complete elimination of autoreactive T cells.

## Two clinically relevant strategies to induce central tolerance in transplant recipients

It is generally recognized that central deletional tolerance provides the most robust long-lasting state of unresponsiveness. Protocols aimed at inducing tolerance through central mechanisms seek to delete alloreactive T cells by "tricking" the recipient's immune system into treating donor antigens as self antigens. In theory, a central strategy requires an intact thymus to select negatively developing recipient T cells with a high affinity for donor antigens. At the same time, the thymus would be expected to educate the developing T cells for a normal repertoire of responses. Based on results from large animal models and some early human studies, there are at least two promising strategies aimed at harnessing the potential of central tolerance in humans—mixed hematopoietic chimerism and donor thymic transplantation.

### Mixed hematopoietic chimerism

This strategy requires a bone marrow or stem cell transplant in addition to the organ transplant. Historically, the experimental transplant recipient has received myeloablative whole-body irradiation to eliminate mature alloreactive T cells and to make "space" for a subsequent donor bone marrow transfusion. Once hematopoietic stem cells contained in the transfusion engraft, they co-exist with recipient stem cells and give rise to cells of all hematopoietic lineages. These donor type cells, along with recipient type cells, seed the thymus and, as described previously, mediate negative selection (Fig. 1). Because cells from the recipient and the donor co-locate to the thymus, self-reactive and donor-reactive T cells are eliminated by negative selection. Consequently, the newly developing T-cell repertoire in mixed chimeras is tolerant toward the donor [8,9].

More recently, a T-cell depleting but non-myeloablative conditioning regimen for the induction of mixed chimerism and tolerance to renal allografts was developed in fully MHC-mismatched cynomolgus monkeys [10]. Elements of the preparative regimen included limited whole-body irradiation plus local thymic supplementation, anti-thymocyte globulin, splenectomy, donor bone marrow cell infusion, and a 1-month posttransplant course of cyclosporine (CsA). Of 13 animals receiving the regimen, 11 developed transient multilineage chimerism, and 9 of these survived long-term. Although transient chimerism appeared essential for the induction of tolerance, peripheral cellular macrochimerism did eventually disappear.

Building upon this success, a case report was published in 2002 describing two patients with end-stage renal disease secondary to multiple myeloma who were treated with simultaneous bone marrow and kidney transplants

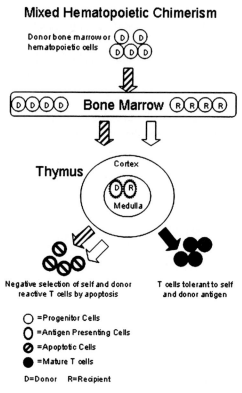

Fig. 1. Development of mixed chimerism via hematopoietic stem cell transplantation. Recipient bone marrow is replaced with donor-derived progenitor cells, and donor and self-reactive T cells undergo negative selection in the recipient thymus, resulting in a T-cell repertoire absent of donor antigen reactivity.

[6]. The bone marrow and kidney, in each case, came from a living-related donor. The recipients received a non-myeloablative conditioning regimen consisting of cyclophosphamide, anti-thymocyte globulin, thymic irradiation, and donor bone marrow infusion followed by CsA for 2 months. In both patients, transient multilineage hematopoietic macrochimerism was induced. Over 5 years later, both patients maintained normal allograft function, were free of signs of acute or chronic rejection, and were off all immunosuppression [6]. The results from this seminal report demonstrate that transplantation tolerance can be induced in the clinical setting.

Because the long-term risk to a patient receiving even a non-myeloablative dose of irradiation is unknown, it is desirable to develop even less toxic protocols for the induction of mixed chimerism. The development of costimulatory-blocking reagents has afforded substantially less toxic mixed chimerism animal protocols. The most frequently used costimulation blockers interfere with the CD28/CTLA4-CD80/CD86 or the CD40L(CD154)-CD40 pathways [11]. Currently, these regimens are being adapted to large animal models so that they may be translated into clinical protocols [12]. If successful, this less toxic conditioning regimen would increase the number of patients considered acceptable for clinical trials.

*Donor thymic transplantation*

Because the thymus mediates the negative selection process [13], it has been suggested that if allogeneic thymic tissue were successfully cotransplanted at the time of organ grafting, it might induce donor-specific tolerance through central deletional mechanisms. The eventual colonization of the transplanted donor thymus with recipient cells would ensure negative selection to both donor and recipient MHC antigens. Although tolerance has been achieved by grafting nonvascularized allogeneic thymic tissue into a variety of host sites in immunodeficient mice [14], efforts to cotransplant nonvascularized thymic tissue at the time of organ transplantation as a means of inducing tolerance in large animals have been unsuccessful. This failure may be due to rejection and loss of the thymic graft before the establishment of adequate vascularization. Indeed, the ischemic period in the first 1 to 3 weeks posttransplant leads to a temporary loss of thymic graft structure, which is reconstituted over the next 5 to 7 weeks [15]. During this period of revascularization, there is an increased susceptibility to nonspecific graft loss and an increased potential for sensitization. This risk may be secondary to the relative difficulty hematopoietic precursors and new thymocytes would have immigrating and emigrating, respectively, from a nonvascularized tissue.

To address the problem of revascularization, novel composite organs called "thymokidneys" [16] and "thymohearts" [17] have been prepared in miniature swine which facilitate the contemporaneous transfer of fully vascularized and functional donor thymic tissue at the time of solid organ transplantation. The thymo-organs are produced by implanting thymic autografts under the renal capsule or epicardium several months before organ harvest. During that time, the thymic tissue undergoes neovascularization, and, when the composite thymo-organ is explanted and grafted, functional vascularized donor thymic tissue is cotransplanted along with the donor organ.

Composite thymokidney grafts have been shown in a swine model to induce tolerance in thymectomized recipients across a class I mismatch barrier with a 12-day course of CsA [18]. All recipients had donor-specific unresponsiveness and no measurable anti-donor antibodies. Additionally, a small percentage of macrochimerism persisted in these animals to at least postoperative day 30. In separate heart allograft studies, thymectomized animals receiving a composite thymoheart demonstrated prolonged allograft survival and diminished development of chronic vascular lesions [19]; however, unlike thymokidney allografts, thymoheart allografts transplanted under a short course of CsA did not induce a state of donor-specific tolerance.

This intolerance was evidenced by the lack of sustained donor-specific unresponsiveness in in vitro assays and the failure to prevent fully cardiac allograft vasculopathy. This difference was probably due to the lesser load of thymic tissue conferred to the host by the thymoheart versus the thymokidney.

To address this issue, Yamada and colleagues [20] have developed a microsurgical technique for vascularized thymic lobe transplantation, and Johnston and coworkers [21] have developed a surgical technique for heart plus en bloc thymus transplantation (Fig. 2). These techniques not only allow more vascularized donor thymus to be conferred to the recipient at the time of organ transplantation but also eliminate the 2- to 3-month period required for thymic neovascularization and thymo-organ creation. Yamada and colleagues reported vascularized thymic lobe induced tolerance and supported thymopoiesis across a fully MHC-mismatched barrier in miniature swine [22]. More recently, they have also demonstrated long-term acceptance of fully mismatched heart grafts without rejection by cotransplantation of vascularized thymic lobe grafts with a short course of immunosuppression [23].

The techniques of vascularized thymic lobe transplantation and en bloc thymus transplantation make the transfer of large amounts of vascularized donor thymus feasible in human recipients with minimal modification of current operative and immunosuppressive regimens. Because of the process of thymic involution, it is believed that donor thymus cotransplantation will be most effective in pediatric and adolescent transplantation.

## Problem 2: there are not enough organs to transplant

Data from the United Network for Organ Sharing indicated that in 2004 there were over 95,000 patients waitlisted for solid organs in the United States but only 27,000 transplants were performed that year [24]. The discrepancy between the number of patients waiting for an organ transplant and the number of organs that become available each year is increasing. For instance, although it is difficult to determine the overall number of patients that would benefit from cardiac transplantation in the United States if the source of donor organs were unlimited, estimates range from 35,000 to 100,000 patients [25]. This scarcity of donor organs has led to a strong resurgence of interest in xenotransplantation over the past decade.

## Solution 2: xenotransplantation

Attempts to salvage dying patients using organ transplants from animals have been attempted before but without success (Table 1). Although many immunologic barriers to xenotransplantation have been identified and overcome, further improvements are necessary before clinical trials can proceed [26].

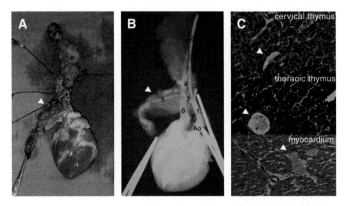

Fig. 2. Arterial anatomy of heart and en bloc thymus grafts. (*A*) Gross specimen of en bloc graft with display of the anterior view of the heart, right cervical thymus (*black arrowhead*), and right thoracic thymus (*white arrowhead*). (*B*) Arterial angiography of en bloc graft performed by means of infusion of barium into the aortic root (Ao). En bloc dissection involves preservation of the innominate artery (1), right carotid artery (2), right axillary artery (3), thyrocervical trunk (4), and right internal thoracic artery (5), as well as fine thymic branches to the cervical (*black arrowhead*) and thoracic (*white arrowhead*) thymic lobes. Venous return is visualized in the superior vena cava (6). (*C*) Hematoxylin and eosin–stained thymus and heart revealed the presence of barium in the small arteries, confirming perfusion. (*From* Johnston DR, Muniappan A, Hoerbelt R, et al. Heart and en bloc thymus transplantation in miniature swine. J Thorac Cardiovasc Surg 2005;130:556; with permission.)

Although the traditional rationale for pursuing xenotransplantation has been its promise to provide an unlimited supply of donor organs, other advantages could be realized by bringing xenotransplantation to the clinic. For instance, by identifying and preparing the donor and recipient in advance of the transplant, the potentially devastating effects of brain death on the donor organ [27] would be eliminated, and the ischemia and reperfusion injury associated with prolonged preservation times [28] would be greatly reduced. There is also the exciting potential for modifying the host and the donor organ before transplantation to not only mitigate the vigorous xenogeneic immune response but also create "customized" donor organs. From an immunologic standpoint, the human recipient may one day be preconditioned is such a way as to induce immunologic tolerance to the xenograft, for instance, by donor bone marrow transplantation [29] or gene therapy [30]. Alternatively, the xenograft could be derived from animals genetically engineered to not express certain harmful gene products (cloned knockout pigs) but to overexpress other beneficial proteins [31]. For instance, right heart dysfunction or failure might be prevented in a donor heart engineered to overexpress SERCA2a (to optimize the use of myocardial calcium), $\beta2$-AR (to improve $\beta$-adrenergic signaling), or Bcl-2 (to block cardiomyocyte apoptosis) [32]. Possibilities such as these add to the enthusiasm for xenotransplantation.

Table 1
World experience in clinical heart xenotransplantation

| Case | Year | Surgeon | Institution | Donor | Type of transplant | Outcome |
|---|---|---|---|---|---|---|
| 1 | 1964 | Hardy | University of Mississippi, Jackson, Mississippi, USA | Chimpanzee | OHT | Functioned 2 h (heart too small to support circulation) |
| 2 | 1968 | Ross | National Heart Hospital, London, UK | Pig | HHT | Cessation of function within 4 min (vascular rejection?) |
| 3 | 1968 | Ross | National Heart Hospital, London, UK | Pig | Perfused with human blood but not transplanted | Immediate cessation of function (vascular rejection?) |
| 4 | 1968 | Cooley | Texas Heart Institute, Houston, Texas, USA | Sheep | OHT | Immediate cessation of function (vascular rejection?) |
| 5 | 1969 | Marion | Lyon, France | Chimpanzee | OHT | Rapid failure (raised pulmonary vascular resistance?) |
| 6 | 1977 | Barnard | University of Capetown, Cape Town, South Africa | Baboon | HHT | Functioned 5 h (heart too small to support circulation) |
| 7 | 1977 | Barnard | University of Capetown, Cape Town, South Africa | Chimpanzee | HHT | Functioned 4 d (failed from probable vascular rejection) |
| 8 | 1984 | Bailey | Loma Linda University, Loma Linda, California, USA | Baboon | OHT | Functioned 20 d (failed from vascular rejection) |
| 9 | 1991 | Religa | Silesian Academy of Medicine, Sosnowiec, Poland | Pig | OHT | Functioned <24 h |
| 10 | 1996 | Baruah | India | Pig | OHT | Functioned <24 h |

*Abbreviations*: HHT, heterotopic heart transplantation; OHT, orthotopic heart transplantation.
*Adapted from* Taniguchi S, Cooper DK. Clinical xenotransplantation: past, present and future. Ann R Coll Surg Eng 1997;79(1):13.

*Choice of animal donor*

Most investigators now believe that the pig will be the most suitable source of organs and tissues for humans. The advantages of swine include unlimited availability, favorable breeding characteristics, and organs that are similar in size and function to their human counterparts (Table 2). Over the last 25 years, a herd of miniature swine has been bred selectively to homozygosity at the porcine MHC [33,34]. These partially inbred miniature swine provide several unique advantages as potential xenograft donors. In contrast to domestic swine that reach 450 kg, adult miniature swine achieve weights of 120 to 140 kg, making it possible to obtain a miniature swine organ of appropriate size for any potential human recipient. A nomogram has been generated relating swine length and human height that predicts the miniature swine that would donate the best size-matched heart for a particular human recipient (Fig. 3) [35].

There are additional advantages to using MHC inbred miniature swine as xenograft donors. Swine have only A and O blood groups, and herds have been bred to be O for the purpose of xenotransplantation donors. From the perspective of genetic engineering, incorporating transgenes into a line of

Table 2
Advantages and disadvantages of baboons and pigs as potential donors of organs and tissue for humans

| Parameter | Baboon | Pig |
| --- | --- | --- |
| Availability | Limited | Unlimited |
| Breeding potential | Poor | Good |
| Period of reproductivity | 3–5 y | 4–8 mo |
| Length of pregnancy | 173–193 d | 112–116 d |
| Number of offspring | 1–2 | 12 (may) |
| Growth | Slow | Rapid[a] |
| Size of adult organs | Inadequate[b] | Adequate |
| Cost of maintenance | High | Significantly lower |
| Anatomic similarity to humans | Close | Moderately close |
| Physiologic similarity to humans | Close | Moderately close |
| Relationship of immune system to humans | Close | Distant |
| Knowledge of tissue typing | Limited | Considerable |
| Necessity for blood type compatibility with humans | Important | Probably unimportant |
| Experience with genetic engineering | None | Considerable |
| Risk of transfer of infection | High | Low |
| Availability of specific pathogen-free animals | None | Yes |
| Public opinion | Mixed | More in favor |

[a] Breeds of miniature swine are approximately 50% of the weight of domestic pigs at birth and sexual maturity, and they reach a maximum weight of approximately 30% of standard breeds.

[b] The size of certain organs (eg, heart) would be inadequate for transplantation into adult humans.

*Adapted from* Cooper DK, Lanza RP. Xeno—the promise of transplanting animal organs into humans. New York: Oxford University Press; 2000.

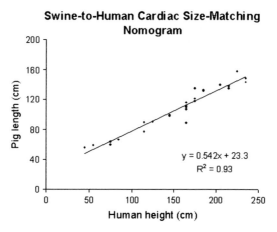

Fig. 3. Swine-to-human cardiac size matching nomogram. The nomogram predicts the best size-matched pig for a prospective human xenograft recipient by matching for aortic annulus diameter. (*From* Allan JS, Rose GA, Choo JK, et al. Morphometric analysis of miniature swine hearts as potential human xenografts. Xenotransplantation 2001;8:92; with permission.)

pigs from the same inbred herd would permit quicker crossbreeding than would be possible if different breeding stocks were used. Although primates may harbor infectious agents such as herpes B virus that can be lethal for human recipients, pigs can be bred to exclude serious human pathogens [36].

*Hyperacute rejection*

The earliest and perhaps most devastating immunologic barrier to xeno-transplantation is hyperacute rejection, which results from the binding of natural antibody to the vascular endothelium of the donor, followed by fix-ation of complement, activation of the endothelium, and, finally, initiation of the coagulation cascade. When a heart is transplanted between discordant species (ie, pig to primate), the once normal-appearing myocardium be-comes dusky and cyanotic, with diminished, if not absent, contractility within minutes of organ reperfusion (Fig. 4). Widespread intravascular thrombosis and interstitial hemorrhage characteristic of a hypercoagulable state mark the histology of this hyperacute rejection response.

Although one might imagine that human natural antibodies would recog-nize a wide array of antigens on pig organs, it has been documented that over 80% of human complement-fixing natural antibodies recognize a single structure, Galα1-3Gal, a carbohydrate that is structurally similar to blood group antigen A and B. The seminal work of Good and Cooper [37,38] and Galili and colleagues [39,40] clearly established the Galα1-3Gal terminal residue (abbreviated as αGal) on pig endothelium as the determinant re-sponsible for binding the major portion of preformed human natural antibodies.

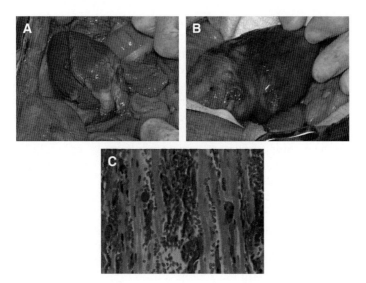

Fig. 4. Hyperacute rejection of swine heart xenograft transplanted into a baboon. (*A*) Photograph taken of a normal pig heart transplanted into the abdomen of an untreated baboon just after the arterial and venous anastomoses are opened and the organ is reperfused. (*B*) Photograph taken 10 minutes after reperfusion of the same pig heart, showing the typical dusky and cyanotic appearance of hyperacute rejection. (*C*) Hematoxylin and eosin–stained micrograph of a myocardial biopsy specimen from the hyperacutely rejected heart xenograft showing interstitial hemorrhage and intravascular thrombosis. (Courtesy of David Cooper, MD, PhD, University of Pittsburgh Medical Center).

## hDAF transgenic swine

Because the complement system results in most of the overt tissue destruction associated with αGal antibodies and hyperacute rejection, the first genetic engineering techniques used to overcome this process targeted pig complement proteins. In humans, the vigor of the complement cascade is regulated by several endothelial proteins, including decay accelerating factor (DAF or CD55), membrane cofactor protein (MCP or CD46), and CD59. These complement regulatory proteins are membrane glycoproteins that act as inhibitors at several key points in the cascade where the activation of both pathways may be halted. Of major importance in discordant xenotransplantation is the fact that these regulatory proteins are effective only with complement proteins of their own species [41]. This concept is the basis for the creation of transgenic animals expressing human complement regulatory proteins.

White and colleagues [42,43] successfully bred transgenic swine that express human delay accelerating factor (hDAF) on their vascular endothelium. When hearts from these hDAF pigs were heterotopically transplanted into nonimmunosuppressed cynomolgus monkeys, hyperacute rejection was successfully avoided. The hDAF hearts survived for up to 5 days (range,

97–126 hours), whereas control hearts from nontransgenic pigs survived for an average of 1.6 days (range, 0.4–101 hours) [44]. Adding pharmacologic immunosuppression (cyclosporine, cyclophosphamide, and methylpredniso-lone) extended hDAF heterotopic cardiac xenograft survival to a median of 40 days [44], with one hDAF heart surviving for 99 days [45]. White and colleagues demonstrated that hearts from hDAF transgenic pigs, orthotopi-cally transplanted into immunosuppressed baboons, were not hyperacutely rejected and maintained adequate cardiac output for 39 days [46,47]. By in-tensifying the immunosuppressive protocol, Kuwaki and colleagues [48] demonstrated the longest survival of a non–life-supporting, pig-to-primate organ to date at 139 days.

Transgenic swine have been produced that express hDAF and human CD59 proteins on their vascular endothelium. Some results suggest that the survival times of hearts from these double transgenic swine do not ex-ceed the survival times of hDAF-expressing hearts [49]. McGregor and col-leagues [50] transplanted hDAF-expressing pig hearts into baboons, but combined the regimen with the administration of a soluble Gal-polythylene glycol conjugate (which removes natural Gal antibody in vivo), T-cell deple-tion, and intense nonspecific immunosuppression. His group achieved xeno-graft heart survival up to 76 days, but the regimen was associated with several infectious complications and posttransplantation lymphoprolifera-tive disorders. The investigators modified the regimen to limit T-cell deple-tion, resulting in one animal surviving 96 days without infectious complications or posttransplantation lymphoproliferative disorders [51].

## Cloned α1,3-Gal knockout pigs

The most effective way to control anti-αGal responses leading to hyper-acute rejection may be to eliminate the gene that encodes for the α1,3GT en-zyme that is necessary for the generation of αGal epitopes. These knockout animals would, by definition, be deficient in αGal epitopes, theoretically leaving no target for human anti-αGal antibodies [52]. Using nuclear trans-fer techniques, healthy piglets have been cloned in which one copy of the α1,3GT gene has been disrupted (heterozygotes) [53,54]. The successful knockout of the α1,3GT locus was confirmed by reverse transcription poly-merase chain reaction (RT-PCR) and southern blot analyses [53]. Since then, homozygote α1,3GT-null pigs have been created that express no αGal epitopes [54].

The development of homozygous α-1,3-galactosyltransferase knockout (GalT-KO) miniature swine offers the exciting prospect of eliminating the devastating barrier of hyperacute rejection [55]. Yamada and coworkers [56] reported the longest life-supporting xenograft to date using the GalT-KO swine as renal xenograft donors to nonhuman primates. By combining GalT-KO kidneys with a treatment regimen aimed at inducing T-cell toler-ance via cotransplantation of vascularized donor thymus, they were able to achieve recipient survival of up to 3 months with stable renal function. These results are even more promising, because at the time of recipient deaths, all combined thymus and kidney recipients had functioning grafts. Of note, baboon recipients of isolated GalT-KO kidney grafts without accompanying thymus rejected the grafts within 34 days [56].

Similar positive results were found with baboon heart transplants [57], but complement fixation and thrombotic microangiopathy resulted in ischemic injury and organ demise (Table 3). Using a regimen based on T-cell depletion and maintenance anti-CD154 monoclonal antibody (mAb) therapy instead of tolerance induction, researchers prevented hyperacute rejection and extended the length of GalT-KO pig heart survival in baboons for up to 6 months. Importantly, this immunosuppressive regimen was associated

Table 3

Therapy, graft survival, and causes of graft failure or death for GalT-KO and GalT-low pig hearts in baboons

| Baboon | CVF (d) | Thymic irradiation (700 cGy) | Antithrombin | Aspirin | Graft survival (d) | Graft failure or death (causes) |
|---|---|---|---|---|---|---|
| Group 1: GalT-KO pig donors (n = 8) | | | | | | |
| B214 | 14 | + | – | – | 59 | TM, focal AHXR, alive |
| B216 | 14 | + | – | – | >56 | Died, heart beating, TM |
| B218 | – | + | – | – | 67 | TM, focal AHXR, alive |
| B223 | – | + | 1–12 | (late) | 110 | MI, TM, AHXR, ACR, vasculopathy, alive |
| B225 | – | + | 1–12 | – | >23 | MI, euthanized, heart beating, minimal TM |
| B226 | 4 | + | – | + | >16 | Euthanized, heart beating, minimal TM |
| B228 | 4 | – | – | + | 179 | TM, focal AHXR, alive |
| B229 | 4 | + | 1–12 | + | 78 | MI, TM, focal AHXR, alive |
| Group 2: GalT-low pig donors (n = 2) | | | | | | |
| B220 | – | + | – | – | <1 | Hyperacute rejection |
| B222 | – | + | – | – | <1 | Hyperacute rejection |

Induction therapy consisted of ATG days −3 to −1, LoCD2b days 1–7, TI day −1, and CVF. Maintenance therapy consisted of anti-human CD154, mycophenolate mofetil, and methylprednisolone. Supportive therapy consisted of ganciclovir, levofloxacin, cometadine, heparin, aspirin, and antithrombin.

*Abbreviations:* ACR, acute cellular rejection; AHXR, acute humoral xenograft rejection; ATG, antithymocyte globulin; CVF, cobra venom factor; LoCD2b, rat anti-human CD2 monoclonal antibody; MI, myocardial infarction; TM, thrombotic microangiopathy.

*Data from* Kuwaki K, Tseng YL, Dor FJ, et al. Heart transplantation in baboons using α 1, 3-galactosyltransferase gene-knockout pigs as donors: initial experience. Nat Med 2005;11(1): 29–31.

with a low incidence of infectious complications or treatment toxicities, demonstrating possible clinical applicability.

To evaluate the efficacy of GalT-KO swine lungs for human lung transplantation, Schroeder and colleagues [58] perfused GalT-KO swine lungs with heparinized human blood. The survival of xenoperfused GalT-KO swine lungs was significantly prolonged in an ex vivo model, but the lungs still showed some evidence of complement fixation and intravascular coagulopathy by the time of graft demise.

## Cellular xenograft rejection

Although great strides have been made in eliminating hyperacute rejection by using organs from GalT-KO swine, controlling T cell–mediated rejection will be essential in bringing xenotransplantation to the clinic. Some of the nonspecific immunosuppressive agents that have been developed to suppress cellular immunity to allografts are likely to have a suppressive effect on the cellular response to discordant xenografts; however, the intensity of immunosuppression that would be required to prevent the rejection of a xenograft would be so great as to make the associated complications of infection, neoplasm, and drug-related side effects intolerable. Indeed, in pig-to-primate xenograft recipients, the high level of immunosuppression required to achieve even moderate survival has resulted in numerous deaths owing to infection and drug-specific complications [47,59]. Many transplant immunologists believe that the success of clinical xenotransplantation will depend on developing ways to induce immunologic tolerance to pig antigens [60]. The two most advanced experimental approaches to inducing T-cell tolerance across a xenograft barrier are mixed chimerism and thymic transplantation.

## Xenogeneic tolerance through mixed chimerism

Based on work in allogeneic systems described previously, the strategy of mixed chimerism has been applied to large animal models of xenotransplantation [29,61]. One such regimen involves depleting mature host T cells by using anti-thymocyte globulin, anti-CD154 mAb, cyclosporine, and mycophenolate mofetil. Large numbers of cytokine-mobilized miniature swine peripheral blood progenitor cells ($3 \times 10^{10}$/kg) are infused at the time of organ transplantation [62] along with species-specific growth factors (pig recombinant stem cell factor and interleukin-3) to promote the survival of the pig cells [63,64]. To prevent antibody-mediated rejection of the porcine hematopoietic cells, extracorporeal immunoadsorption of anti-Gal antibodies [65–68], in addition to cobra venom factor and host splenectomy, have been employed [69,70].

Using this regimen, porcine cells have been detectable in conditioned baboons on occasion for over 20 days by flow cytometry and for at least 1 month by PCR [71,72]. Invariably, there was a return of anti-αGal antibodies, which coincided with loss of the pig cells. This return precluded subsequent organ transplantation. Current efforts are focusing on attempts to increase the engraftment of porcine hematopoietic progenitor cells in primate recipients by including strategies aimed at effectively eliminating or suppressing anti-αGal antibodies.

*Xenogeneic tolerance through thymic transplantation*

The difficulty in coercing xenogeneic hematopoietic cells to migrate to the recipient thymus and induce deletional tolerance through a strategy of mixed chimerism might be overcome by replacing the recipient thymus with the thymus from the xenogeneic organ donor after host T-cell depletion and thymectomy. Support for this notion comes from studies in which thymectomized, T cell–depleted mice transplanted with discordant pig thymic grafts not only demonstrated functional recovery of murine CD4 T cells in the pig thymic grafts [73,74] but became tolerant to donor xenogeneic skin grafts [75].

Efforts to extend thymus xenografting to the pig-to-primate model have achieved partial success. Thymectomized baboons treated with an anti-CD3 mAb immunotoxin to deplete pre-existing peripheral T cells showed transient engraftment of porcine thymic tissue. Furthermore, they demonstrated specific in vitro unresponsiveness to the pig donor while maintaining full alloresponsiveness and exhibited prolonged donor-specific skin graft survival [76,77]. These results suggest that strategies to improve pig thymus engraftment may have the potential to achieve T-cell tolerance in primates [61].

*Infectious disease obstacles*

The possibility that an animal organ donor will pass an infectious agent (xenozoonoses) to a human xenograft recipient and that the infection may be passed to the human population in general has been the center of much debate [78,79]. On the one hand, transplanting a pig organ into a human patient bypasses many natural defenses or barriers to infection. Furthermore, the immunosuppression required to prevent xenograft rejection may result in a further reduction in the host's resistance to infections. Most concern has revolved around the transfer of porcine endogenous retroviruses (PERVs) [80,81]. These retroviruses are similar to human endogenous retroviruses (HERVs), which are present in all human cells. Recent data have shown that PERVs can infect human cells in vitro [82].

No known passage of PERVs to humans has ever occurred in vivo, and no human disease associated with PERVs (or for that matter HERVs) has ever been observed [83]. Using gnotobiotic (germ free or animals with a defined microbial composition) techniques of delivering piglets, early weaning from the sow, and pathogen-free housing facilities may result in pigs actually representing less of an infectious threat than the current human donor pool for hearts, which frequently carries cytomegalovirus and Epstein-Barr virus, as well as hepatitis and HIV [25,84,85].

Although it is generally believed that the potential for infectious risk associated with successful xenotransplantation is low, knowledge regarding known and novel xenozoonoses must be expanded. For further information, the reader is referred to two excellent reviews [25,86].

## Summary

Achieving transplantation tolerance will have enormous benefits for current recipients of allogeneic grafts and future recipients of xenogeneic grafts. Our sophistication in developing clinically relevant tolerance induction protocols is increasing in proportion to our understanding of the barriers that still remain in the way of the consistent induction of a tolerant state.

## Acknowledgments

The authors thank Dr. Kazuhiko Yamada for his critical review of this manuscript.

## References

[1] Taylor DO, Edwards LB, Boucek MM, et al. The Registry of the International Society for Heart and Lung Transplantation: twenty-first official adult heart transplant report–2004. J Heart Lung Transplant 2004;23:796–803.

[2] Merion RM. Preface: 2003 SRTR Report on the State of Transplantation. Am J Transplant 2004;4(Suppl 9):5–6.

[3] Billingham RE, Brent L, Medawar PB. Actively acquired tolerance to foreign cells. Nature 1953;172:603–6.

[4] Auchincloss H Jr. In search of the elusive Holy Grail: the mechanisms and prospects for achieving clinical transplantation tolerance. Am J Transplant 2001;1:6–12.

[5] Spitzer TR, Delmonico F, Tolkoff-Rubin N, et al. Combined histocompatibility leukocyte antigen-matched donor bone marrow and renal transplantation for multiple myeloma with end stage renal disease: the induction of allograft tolerance through mixed lymphohematopoietic chimerism. Transplantation 1999;68:480–4.

[6] Buhler LH, Spitzer TR, Sykes M, et al. Induction of kidney allograft tolerance after transient lymphohematopoietic chimerism in patients with multiple myeloma and end-stage renal disease. Transplantation 2002;74:1405–9.

[7] Waldmann H, Graca L, Cobbold S, et al. Regulatory T cells and organ transplantation. Semin Immunol 2004;16:119–26.

[8] Wekerle T, Sykes M. Mixed chimerism as an approach for the induction of transplantation tolerance. Transplantation 1999;68:459–67.

[9] Ildstad ST, Sachs DH. Reconstitution with syngeneic plus allogeneic or xenogeneic bone marrow leads to specific acceptance of allografts or xenografts. Nature 1984;307:168–70.

[10] Kawai T, Cosimi AB, Colvin RB, et al. Mixed allogeneic chimerism and renal allograft tolerance in cynomolgus monkeys. Transplantation 1995;59:256–62.

[11] Wekerle T, Sykes M. Induction of tolerance. Surgery 2004;135:359–64.

[12] Kawai T, Sachs DH, Cosimi AB. Tolerance to vascularized organ allografts in large-animal models. Curr Opin Immunol 1999;11:516–20.

[13] Hoffmann MW, Allison J, Miller JFAP. Tolerance induction by thymic medullary epithelium. Proc Natl Acad Sci USA 1992;89:2526–30.
[14] Waer M, Palathumpat V, Sobis H, et al. Induction of transplantation tolerance in mice across major histocompatibility barrier by using allogeneic thymus transplantation and total lymphoid irradiation. J Immunol 1990;145:499–504.
[15] Haller GW, Esnaola N, Yamada K, et al. Thymic transplantation across an MHC class I barrier in swine. J Immunol 1999;163:3785–92.
[16] Yamada K, Shimizu A, Ierino FL, et al. Thymic transplantation in miniature swine. I. Development and function of the "thymokidney". Transplantation 1999;68:1684–92.
[17] Lambrigts D, Menard MT, Alexandre GPJ, et al. Creation of the "thymoheart" allograft: implantation of autologous thymus into the heart prior to procurement. Transplantation 1998;66:810–4.
[18] Yamada K, Shimizu A, Utsugi R, et al. Thymic transplantation in miniature swine. II. Induction of tolerance by transplantation of composite thymokidneys to thymectomized recipients. J Immunol 2000;164:3079–86.
[19] Menard MT, Schwarze ML, Allan JS, et al. Composite "thymoheart" transplantation improves cardiac allograft survival. Am J Transplant 2004;4:79–86.
[20] LaMattina JC, Kumagai N, Barth RN, et al. Vascularized thymic lobe transplantation in miniature swine. I. Vascularized thymic lobe allografts support thymopoiesis. Transplantation 2002;73:826–31.
[21] Johnston DR, Muniappan A, Hoerbelt R, et al. Heart and en-bloc thymus transplantation in miniature swine. J Thorac Cardiovasc Surg 2005;130:554–9.
[22] Kamano C, Vagefi PA, Kumagai N, et al. Vascularized thymic lobe transplantation in miniature swine: thymopoiesis and tolerance induction across fully MHC-mismatched barriers. Proc Natl Acad Sci USA 2004;101:3827–32.
[23] Nobori S, Samelson-Jones E, Shimizu A, et al. Long-term acceptance of fully allogeneic cardiac grafts by cotransplantation of vascularized thymus in miniature swine. Transplantation 2006;81:26–35.
[24] UNOS. Waiting list data: 2001. United Network for Organ Sharing 2001. Available at: http://www.unos.org. Accessed April 2006.
[25] Cooper DKC, Keogh AM, Brink J, et al. Report of the Xenotransplantation Advisory Committee of the International Society for Heart and Lung Transplantation: the present status of xenotransplantation and its potential role in the treatment of end-stage cardiac and pulmonary diseases. J Heart Lung Transplant 2000;19:1125–65.
[26] Yamada K, Griesemer A, Okumi M. Pigs as xenogenic donors. Transplant Rev 2005;19:164–77.
[27] Pratschke J, Wilhelm MJ, Kusaka M, et al. Brain death and its influence on donor organ quality and outcome after transplantation. Transplantation 1999;67:343–8.
[28] Laskowski I, Pratschke J, Wilhelm MJ, et al. Molecular and cellular events associated with ischemia/reperfusion injury. Ann Transplant 2000;5:29–35.
[29] Sykes M, Sachs DH. Mixed chimerism. Philos Trans R Soc Lond B Biol Sci 2001;356:707–26.
[30] Bracy JL, Sachs DH, Iacomini J. Inhibition of xenoreactive natural antibody production by retroviral gene therapy. Science 1998;281:1845–7.
[31] Salama AD, Delikouras A, Pusey CD, et al. Transplant accommodation in highly sensitized patients: a potential role of Bcl-xL and alloantibody. Am J Transplant 2001;1:260–9.
[32] Hajjar RJ, del Monte F, Matsui T, et al. Prospects for gene therapy for heart failure. Circ Res 2000;86:616–21.
[33] Sachs DH. MHC homozygous miniature swine. In: Swindle MM, Moody DC, Phillips LD, editors. Swine as models in biomedical research. Ames (IA): Iowa State University Press; 1992. p. 3–15.
[34] Sachs DH. The pig as a potential xenograft donor. Pathol Biol 1994;42:217–28.

[35] Allan JS, Rose GA, Choo JK, et al. Morphometric analysis of miniature swine hearts as potential human xenografts. Xenotransplantation 2001;8:90–3.

[36] Fishman JA. Infection and xenotransplantation: developing strategies to minimize risk. Ann N Y Acad Sci 1998;862:52–66.

[37] Good AH, Cooper DKC, Malcolm AJ, et al. Identification of carbohydrate structures that bind human antiporcine antibodies: implications for discordant xenografting in humans. Transplant Proc 1992;24:559–62.

[38] Cooper DKC, Good AH, Koren E, et al. Identification of alpha-galactosyl and other carbohydrate epitopes that are bound by human anti-pig antibodies: relevance to discordant xenografting in man. Transpl Immunol 1993;1:198–205.

[39] Galili U, Macher BA, Buehler J, et al. Human natural anti-$\alpha$-galactosyl IgG. II. The specific recognition of $\alpha$(1-3) linked galactose residues. J Exp Med 1985;162:573–82.

[40] Galili U, Rachmilewitz EA, Peleg A, et al. A unique natural human IgG antibody with anti-alpha-galactosyl specificity. J Exp Med 1984;160:1519–31.

[41] Dalmasso AP, Vercelolotti GM, Platt JL, et al. Inhibition of complement-mediated endothelial cell cytotoxicity by decay-accelerating factor: potential for prevention of xenograft hyperacute rejection. Transplantation 1991;52:530–3.

[42] Cozzi E, White DJG. The generation of transgenic pigs as potential organs donors for humans. Nat Med 1995;1:964–6.

[43] Schmoeckel M, Nollert G, Shahmohammadi M, et al. Prevention of hyperacute rejection by human decay accelerating factor in xenogeneic perfused working hearts. Transplantation 1996;62:729–34.

[44] Cozzi E, Yannoutsos N, Langford GA, et al. Effect of transgenic expression of human decay-accelerating factor on the inhibition of hyperacute rejection of pig organs. In: Cooper DKC, Kemp E, Platt JL, et al, editors. Xenotransplantation. Heidelberg: Springer-Verlag; 1997. p. 665–82.

[45] Bhatti FN, Schmoeckel M, Zaidi A, et al. Three-month survival of HDAFF transgenic pig hearts transplanted into primates. Transplant Proc 1999;31:958.

[46] Vial CM, Ostlie DJ, Bhatti FN, et al. Life supporting function for over one month of a transgenic porcine heart in a baboon. J Heart Lung Transplant 2000;19(2):224–9.

[47] Schmoeckel M, Bhatti FNK, Zaidi A, et al. Orthotopic heart transplantation in a transgenic pig-to-primate model. Transplantation 1998;65:1570–7.

[48] Kuwaki K, Knosalla C, Dor FJMF, et al. Suppression of natural and elicited antibodies in pig-to-baboon heart transplantation using a human anti-human CD154 mAb-based regimen. Am J Transplant 2004;4(3):363–72.

[49] Byrne GW, McCurry KR, Martin MJ, et al. Transgenic pigs expressing human CD59 and decay-accelerating factor produce an intrinsic barrier to complement-mediated damage. Transplantation 1997;63:149–55.

[50] McGregor CG, Teotia SS, Schirmer JM, et al. Advances in preclinical cardiac xenotransplantation. J Heart Lung Transplant 2003;22:S89.

[51] McGregor CG, Davies WR, Oi K, et al. Cardiac xenotransplantation: recent preclinical progress with 3-month median survival. J Thorac Cardiovasc Surg 2005;130:844–51.

[52] Cooper DKC, Koren E, Oriol R. Genetically engineered pigs. Lancet 1993;342:682–3.

[53] Dai Y, Vaught TD, Boone J, et al. Targeted disruption of the alpha-1,3-galactosyltransferase gene in cloned pigs. Nat Biotechnol 2002;20:251–5.

[54] Lai L, Kolber-Simonds D, Park KW, et al. Production of alpha-1,3-galactosyltransferase knockout pigs by nuclear transfer cloning. Science 2002;295:1089–92.

[55] Kolber-Simonds D, Lai L, Watt SR, et al. Production of alpha-1,3-galactosyltransferase null pigs by means of nuclear transfer with fibroblasts bearing loss of heterozygosity mutations. Proc Natl Acad Sci USA 2004;101:7335–40.

[56] Yamada K, Yazawa K, Shimizu A, et al. Marked prolongation of porcine renal xenograft survival in baboons through the use of alpha-1,3-galactosyltransferase gene-knockout donors and the cotransplantation of vascularized thymic tissue. Nat Med 2005;11:32–4.

[57] Kuwaki K, Tseng YL, Dor FJ, et al. Heart transplantation in baboons using alpha-1,3-galactosyltransferase gene-knockout pigs as donors: initial experience. Nat Med 2005;11:29–31.
[58] Schroeder C, Allan JS, Nguyen B-N, et al. Hyperacute rejection is attenuated in GalT-KO swine lungs perfused ex vivo with human blood. Transplant Proc 2005;37(1):512–3.
[59] Zaidi A, Schmoeckel M, Bhatti F, et al. Life-supporting pig-to-primate renal xenotransplantation using genetically modified donors. Transplantation 1998;65:1584–90.
[60] Dorling A, Lechler RI. T cell–mediated xenograft rejection: specific tolerance is probably required for long term xenograft survival. Xenotransplantation 1998;5:234–45.
[61] Sachs DH, Sykes M, Robson SC, et al. Xenotransplantation. In: Dixon FJ, editor. Advances in immunology. San Diego: Academic Press; 2001. p. 129–233.
[62] Buhler L, Awwad M, Basker M, et al. High-dose porcine hematopoietic cell transplantation combined with CD40 ligand blockade in baboons prevents an induced anti-pig humoral response. Transplantation 2000;69:2296–304.
[63] Alexandre GPJ, Squifflet JP, deBruyere M, et al. Present experiences in a series of 26 ABO-incompatible living donor renal allografts. Transplant Proc 1987;19:4538.
[64] Sachs DH, Sablinski T. Tolerance across discordant xenogeneic barriers. Xenotransplantation 1995;2:234–9.
[65] Latinne D, Smith CV, Nickeleit V, et al. Xenotransplantation from pig to cynomolgus monkey: approach toward tolerance induction. Transplant Proc 1993;25:336.
[66] Tanaka M, Latinne D, Sablinski T, et al. Xenotransplantation from pig to cynomolgus monkey: the potential for overcoming xenograft rejection through induction of chimerism. Transplant Proc 1994;26:1326.
[67] Sablinski T, Latinne D, Bailin M, et al. Xenotransplantation of pig kidneys to nonhuman primates. I. Development of the model. Xenotransplantation 1995;2:264–70.
[68] Sachs DH, Sykes M, Greenstein J, et al. Tolerance and xenograft survival. Nat Med 1995;1(9):969.
[69] Xu Y, Lorf T, Sablinski T, et al. Removal of anti-porcine natural antibodies from human and nonhuman primate plasma in vitro and in vivo by a Galα1–3Galβ1–4βGlc-X immunoaffinity column. Transplantation 1998;65:172–9.
[70] Kozlowski T, Fuchimoto Y, Monroy R, et al. Apheresis and column absorption for specific removal of Gal-alpha-1, 3 Gal natural antibodies in a pig-to-baboon model. Transplant Proc 1997;29:961.
[71] Buhler L, Awwad M, Treter S, et al. Induction of mixed hematopoietic chimerism in the pig-to-baboon model. Transplant Proc 2000;32:1101.
[72] Buhler L, Basker M, Alwayn IP, et al. Coagulation and thrombotic disorders associated with pig organ and hematopoietic cell transplantation in nonhuman primates. Transplantation 2000;70:1323–31.
[73] Lee LA, Gritsch HA, Sergio JJ, et al. Specific tolerance across a discordant xenogeneic transplantation barrier. Proc Natl Acad Sci USA 1994;91:10864–7.
[74] Zhao Y, Fishman JA, Sergio JJ, et al. Immune restoration by fetal pig thymus grafts in T cell–depleted, thymectomized mice. J Immunol 1997;158:1641–9.
[75] Zhao Y, Swenson K, Sergio JJ, et al. Skin graft tolerance across a discordant xenogeneic barrier. Nat Med 1996;2:1211–6.
[76] Wu A, Yamada K, Awwad M, et al. Effects of xenogeneic thymic transplantation in baboons. Transplant Proc 2001;33:766.
[77] Wu A, Yamada K, Awwad M, et al. Experience with porcine thymic transplantation in baboons. Transplant Proc 2000;32:1048.
[78] Bach FH, Fineberg HV. Call for moratorium on xenotransplants. Nature 1998;391:326.
[79] Sachs DH, Colvin RB, Cosimi AB, et al. Xenotransplantation–caution, but no moratorium. Nat Med 1998;4:372–3.
[80] Stoye JP, Coffin JM. The dangers of xenotransplantation. Nat Med 1995;1:1100.
[81] Patience C, Takeuchi Y, Weiss RA. Zoonosis in xenotransplantation. Curr Opin Immunol 1998;10:539–42.

[82] Patience C, Takeuchi Y, Weiss RA. Infection of human cells by an endogenous retrovirus of pigs. Nat Med 1997;3:282–6.

[83] Paradis K, Langford G, Long Z, et al. Search for cross-species transmission of porcine endogenous retrovirus in patients treated with living pig tissue: the XEN 111 Study Group. Science 1999;285:1236–41.

[84] Cooper DK, Keogh AM, Brink J, et al. Report of the Xenotransplantation Advisory Committee of the International Society for Heart and Lung Transplantation: the present status of xenotransplantation and its potential role in the treatment of end-stage cardiac and pulmonary diseases. J Heart Lung Transplant 2000;19:1125–65.

[85] Onions D, Cooper DK, Alexander TJ, et al. An approach to the control of disease transmission in pig-to-human xenotransplantation. Xenotransplantation 2000;7:143–55.

[86] Fishman JA. Xenosis and xenotransplantation: addressing the infectious risks posed by an emerging technology. Kidney Int Suppl 1997;58:S41–5.

ELSEVIER
SAUNDERS

SURGICAL
CLINICS OF
NORTH AMERICA

Surg Clin N Am 86 (2006) 1297–1304

# Index

*Note:* Page numbers of article titles are in **boldface** type.

# Moving?

## Make sure your subscription moves with you!

To notify us of your new address, find your **Clinics Account Number** (located on your mailing label above your name), and contact customer service at:

**E-mail: elspcs@elsevier.com**

**800-654-2452** (subscribers in the U.S. & Canada)
**407-345-4000** (subscribers outside of the U.S. & Canada)

**Fax number: 407-363-9661**

**Elsevier Periodicals Customer Service**
6277 Sea Harbor Drive
Orlando, FL 32887-4800

*To ensure uninterrupted delivery of your subscription, please notify us at least 4 weeks in advance of move.

United States Postal Service

## Statement of Ownership, Management, and Circulation

| 1. Publication Title | 2. Publication Number | 3. Filing Date |
|---|---|---|
| Surgical Clinics of North America | 5 2 9 - 8 0 0 0 | 9/15/06 |

| 4. Issue Frequency | 5. Number of Issues Published Annually | 6. Annual Subscription Price |
|---|---|---|
| Feb, Apr, Jun, Aug, Oct, Dec | 6 | $200.00 |

**7.** Complete Mailing Address of Known Office of Publication (Not printer) (Street, city, county, state, and ZIP+4)

Elsevier Inc.
360 Park Avenue South
New York, NY 10010-1710

Contact Person
Sarah Carmichael

Telephone
(215) 239-3681

**8.** Complete Mailing Address of Headquarters or General Business Office of Publisher (Not printer)

Elsevier Inc., 360 Park Avenue South, New York, NY 10010-1710

**9.** Full Names and Complete Mailing Addresses of Publisher, Editor, and Managing Editor (Do not leave blank)

Publisher (Name and complete mailing address)

John Schrefer, Elsevier Inc., 1600 John F. Kennedy Blvd., Suite 1800, Philadelphia, PA 19103-2899

Editor (Name and complete mailing address)

Catherine Bewick, Elsevier Inc., 1600 John F. Kennedy Blvd., Suite 1800, Philadelphia, PA 19103-2899

Managing Editor (Name and complete mailing address)

Catherine Bewick, Elsevier Inc., 1600 John F. Kennedy Blvd., Suite 1800, Philadelphia, PA 19103-2899

**10.** Owner (Do not leave blank. If the publication is owned by a corporation, give the name and address of the corporation immediately followed by the names and addresses of all stockholders owning or holding 1 percent or more of the total amount of stock. If not owned by a corporation, give the names and addresses of the individual owners. If owned by a partnership or other unincorporated firm, give its name and address as well as those of each individual owner. If the publication is published by a nonprofit organization, give its name and address.)

| Full Name | Complete Mailing Address |
|---|---|
| Wholly owned subsidiary of | 4520 East-West Highway |
| Reed/Elsevier Inc., US holdings | Bethesda, MD 20814 |

**11.** Known Bondholders, Mortgagees, and Other Security Holders Owning or Holding 1 Percent or More of Total Amount of Bonds, Mortgages, or Other Securities. If none, check box ▶ ☐ None

| Full Name | Complete Mailing Address |
|---|---|
| N/A | |

**12.** Tax Status (For completion by nonprofit organizations authorized to mail at nonprofit rates) (Check one)
The purpose, function, and nonprofit status of this organization and the exempt status for federal income tax purposes:
☐ Has Not Changed During Preceding 12 Months
☐ Has Changed During Preceding 12 Months (Publisher must submit explanation of change with this statement)

(See Instructions on Reverse)

PS Form **3526**, October 1999

| 13. Publication Title | | | | 14. Issue Date for Circulation Data Below |
|---|---|---|---|---|
| Surgical Clinics of North America | | | | June 2006 |

| 15. | Extent and Nature of Circulation | | | Average No. Copies Each Issue During Preceding 12 Months | No. Copies of Single Issue Published Nearest to Filing Date |
|---|---|---|---|---|---|
| a. | Total Number of Copies (Net press run) | | | 6,417 | 5,800 |
| b. Paid and/or Requested Circulation | | (1) | Paid/Requested Outside-County Mail Subscriptions Stated on Form 3541. (Include advertiser's proof and exchange copies) | 3,138 | 2,716 |
| | | (2) | Paid In-County Subscriptions Stated on Form 3541 (Include advertiser's proof and exchange copies) | | |
| | | (3) | Sales Through Dealers and Carriers, Street Vendors, Counter Sales, and Other Non-USPS Paid Distribution | 2,090 | 2,042 |
| | | (4) | Other Classes Mailed Through the USPS | | |
| c. | Total Paid and/or Requested Circulation [Sum of 15b. (1), (2), (3), and (4)] | | ▶ | 5,228 | 4,758 |
| d. Free Distribution by Mail (Samples, complimentary, and other free) | | (1) | Outside-County as Stated on Form 3541 | 245 | 224 |
| | | (2) | In-County as Stated on Form 3541 | | |
| | | (3) | Other Classes Mailed Through the USPS | | |
| e. | Free Distribution Outside the Mail (Carriers or other means) | | ▶ | 245 | 224 |
| f. | Total Free Distribution (Sum of 15d. and 15e.) | | ▶ | | |
| g. | Total Distribution (Sum of 15c. and 15f.) | | ▶ | 5,473 | 4,982 |
| h. | Copies not Distributed | | | 943 | 818 |
| i. | Total (Sum of 15g. and h.) | | ▶ | 6,417 | 5,800 |
| j. | Percent Paid and/or Requested Circulation (15c. divided by 15g. times 100) | | | 95.52% | 95.50% |

**16.** Publication of Statement of Ownership
☐ Publication required. Will be printed in the **October 2006** issue of this publication. ☐ Publication not required

**17.** Signature and Title of Editor, Publisher, Business Manager, or Owner

*John Fanucci* – Executive Director of Subscription Services

Date 9/15/06

I certify that all information furnished on this form is true and complete. I understand that anyone who furnishes false or misleading information on this form or who omits material or information requested on the form may be subject to criminal sanctions (including fines and imprisonment) and/or civil sanctions (including civil penalties).

### Instructions to Publishers

1. Complete and file one copy of this form with your postmaster annually on or before October 1. Keep a copy of the completed form for your records.
2. In cases where the stockholder or security holder is a trustee, include in items 10 and 11 the name of the person or corporation for whom the trustee is acting. Also include the names and addresses of individuals who are stockholders who own or hold 1 percent or more of the total amount of bonds, mortgages, or other securities of the publishing corporation. In item 11, if none, check the box. Use blank sheets if more space is required.
3. Be sure to furnish all circulation information called for in item 15. Free circulation must be shown in items 15d, e, and f.
4. Item 15h., Copies not Distributed, must include (1) newsstand copies originally stated on Form 3541, and returned to the publisher, (2) estimated returns from news agents, and (3), copies for office use, leftovers, spoiled, and all other copies not distributed.
5. If the publication had Periodicals authorization as a general or requester publication, this Statement of Ownership, Management, and Circulation must be published; it must be printed in any issue in October or, if the publication is not published during October, the first issue printed after October.
6. In item 16, indicate the date of the issue in which this Statement of Ownership will be published.
7. Item 17 must be signed.

*Failure to file or publish a statement of ownership may lead to suspension of Periodicals authorization.*

PS Form **3526**, October 1999 (Reverse)